The 5 PRINCIPLES of AGELESS LIVING

Also by Dayle Haddon

Ageless Beauty: A Woman's Guide to
Lifelong Beauty and Well-Being

The *The* 5 PRINCIPLES *of* AGELESS LIVING

A Woman's Guide to Lifelong Health, Beauty, and Well-Being

DAYLE HADDON

ATRIA BOOKS

New York   London   Toronto   Sydney

PLEASE NOTE: I hope this book proves helpful in your life. However, the information contained herein is not intended to replace medical advice or to be a substitute for a physician. Always seek the advice of a physician before beginning any diet and/or exercise program.

The author and the publisher expressly disclaim responsibility for any adverse effects arising from following advice in this book without appropriate medical supervision.

A ATRIA BOOKS

1230 Avenue of the Americas
New York, NY 10020

ISBN: 0-7434-6341-2
      0-7432-4325-0 (Pbk)

First Atria Books trade paperback edition May 2005

10   9   8   7   6   5   4   3   2

ATRIA BOOKS is a trademark of Simon & Schuster, Inc.

Manufactured in the United States of America

For information regarding special discounts for bulk purchases, please contact Simon & Schuster Special Sales at 1-800-456-6798 or business@simonandschuster.com

Excerpt from *A Return to Love* by Marianne Williamson (HarperCollins, 1996), reprinted with permission.

To my daughter, Ryan, who taught me about love.

I delighted in the child you were,

and take pride in seeing the wise woman you are becoming.

I'm glad to share this glorious journey with you.

Acknowledgments

There are so many people who have helped bring this book into being. I could not have done it without them. First, I must thank my loving family, which has always given me the support and love to dare. My daughter, her husband, and my grandchildren, who are and continue to be a source of joy and wonder for me. The undaunting spirit of my editor, Brenda Copeland, whose commitment, vision, and all-embracing passion made working with her a complete pleasure. Judith Curr, publisher of Atria Books, who immediately understood the message of this book and who shepherded it through with caring hands; and to Seale Ballenger and Louise Braverman for their enthusiasm and energy. Thank you.

To Pam Janis, who sorted through all the information with me, helping me find the most important messages with such enthusiasm, laughter, and tears: thank you for the shared adventure. To Dominick Kulik and Shannon Box Kulik, the godparents of this project for their unwavering belief, steadfast work, and shared vision to uplift, thank you.

Thank you from the bottom of my heart to my dear friends, who have no idea of the treasures they give me every day by their presence, and who supported me all through my absence as I wrote this book for the last year: to Michele, Regina, Elisabeth, Christine, Barbara, and Jennifer, and to the Froggy Club—Deb, Carole, and Mary Lou.

Thank you to Lindsey Owen-Jones, Patrick Rabain, and Nicholas Hieronimus for your extraordinary grace and conviction. To Jean Paul Agon, Joe Campinell, and Carol Hamilton for your vision and commitment. And to everyone I've worked so closely with at L'Oréal worldwide—thank you for all the wonderful things you do.

Thanks for the constant support of Linda Hann, who kept the ball rolling, and my thanks for the extra help from dermatologists Katie Rodan, Amy Lewis, and Lydia Evans.

Thank you to Cheryl Richardson for her kind words, and for her constant commitment to women.

A special thank-you to my dear friend Reece, whose patience, care, support, and love are an inspiring example to me every day. His unwavering enthusiasm for this book from the very beginning gave me so much.

And lastly, I would like to thank the women whose courage, insight, and innate sense of joy create balance and harmony for all of us.

It is never too late to be what you might have been.

—GEORGE ELIOT

CONTENTS

Foreword XIII

Preface XVII

The Adventure
1

The Principles
19

Principle One: Look Your Best
25

Principle Two: Nurture Your Spirit
91

Principle Three: Honor Your Body
139

Principle Four: Discover Your Wisdom
205

Principle Five: Stay Connected
257

The Adventure Continues . . .
305

Ageless Living Dialogue
311

Midlife Myths and Maxims
319

Resource Guide 321

Index 339

Foreword

Dear Reader,

Midlife is a time of introspection and evaluation when we look back at the choices we've made that have brought us to this point in our lives. For some women, it serves as a time of celebration—a reason to feel good about the way you've lived your life. For others, it's a time of frustration and fear—fear that the life you truly want to live will become less and less possible with each passing year. If this rings true for you, don't worry, you're not alone. Most women feel as though the lives they live do not reflect their deepest longings and desires. It's important to remember this: you have a choice about how you spend each and every moment of your precious life. You can begin, right now, to take small steps that will allow you to join the ranks of women who are celebrating ageless living!

When it comes to getting older, I've been lucky. My close (older) friends have always celebrated aging. At birthday gatherings I hear them say things like: "Life only gets better with age!" Or, "The older I get, the stronger I feel. Now I care more about what *I* think instead of what everyone else thinks." These messages have deeply influenced the way I view getting older. Rather than fear the passing of time, I feel a sense of excited anticipation with the approach of every new year. The power of positive role models has helped me form beliefs about aging that have served me in empowering ways. I always know in my heart that the next year of my life will provide me with the wisdom and experience to live a happier and healthier life. And it has . . .

The year I turned forty, I met Dayle Haddon. We were introduced to each other at an event in Santa Fe, New Mexico, where we were both scheduled to speak. As I listened to Dayle share her life story, I was impressed by her incredible grace and power. She had been challenged by some of life's most difficult circumstances—the death of a husband, the need to reenter the workforce after years of raising a child, and the stress and conflict that can arise when women try to achieve success in their professional life, while honoring their high standards of parenting a child. It was obvious that the difficulties Dayle faced had only served to make her stronger and wiser.

During lunch, Dayle and I had a chance to talk. Immediately she felt like a kindred spirit. She had a deep commitment to self-care and it showed. She radiated beauty—a deep, soulful beauty that comes from living with integrity. Dayle has that rare quality of "congruence"— someone who walks her talk, and honors her whole self— body, mind and spirit. It's this quality of authenticity and inner beauty that makes her the perfect person to write a book about ageless living.

If you're ready to enter the next phase of your life with a sense of excitement and anticipation, you'll want to read (and use!) the practical advice and resources offered in this book. As a warm and compassionate guide, Dayle will show you why beauty, true beauty, starts on the inside with the relationship you form with yourself. She'll share her simple, step-by-step process for looking your best, honoring your self-care, uncovering the wisdom you've gained from years of life experience, and using it to create deeper connections with those you love.

Now more than ever the world needs healthy, whole, vibrant women who own their grace and power. I urge you to give yourself the gift of this book. As you honor your needs by using Dayle's five principles for ageless living, you'll begin to see that the process of aging presents you with the opportunity to experience a beautiful unfolding of your most authentic self. Enjoy!

Cheryl Richardson

Preface

If someone had asked me fifteen years ago to write a book about ageless living, I wouldn't have known where to begin. I was living in France at the time, and I was happy and comfortable. My life was fairly typical for a mother in her late thirties who had had a successful career and was juggling the day-to-day responsibilities of running a household, caring for a husband, and mothering a teenage daughter. Life was good. Then, in an instant, it turned upside down. My husband died. I had few resources to fall back on. I was struggling to do the best I could as a single parent and I needed to find work. I was devastated. I never thought I'd make it.

This book comes from things I've learned during the last fifteen years, both from my own experience and from observing others. Not every woman has a close death in her family or finds herself unexpectedly back in the job market, frightened and unprepared. But we all have challenges and hardships, and we all go through changes, especially at midlife. I have been thinking about many of the concepts in this book for a lifetime, but they all seem to have come together for me now. The ideas of triumph in the face of challenge and living a better life—a *true* life—have been talked about by others. I don't claim to have invented these notions, but I have thought a great deal about what it means to live true to myself. I've had to. I've thought about happiness and I've thought about faith. I've thought about age. I've thought about purpose and service, and about all the things that make us great or small. What makes these ideas so important to me is that as I hit my forties, and now my fifties, I see that they are not only needed to drag someone out of a hole, as I was in, but that they are also essential to anyone who wants to live a big, fabulous, true life.

After my husband died I felt I would never be able to come up for air. Not only did I lose my partner, I lost my home and all of my savings. Even though I had worked since I was a teenager, I was shocked to find that through ignorance on my part and mismanagement by others, there was nothing left. I had no work possibilities and, at the time, nowhere to turn. Everything looked bleak. But I had my health. And I had my daughter. My biggest concern, Ryan became the fire beneath me, my reason to get back on track. How was I going to support her? How was I going to find us a home or put her through school? I didn't know where to start. But I knew I had to try. I had no other choice.

It was only by traveling through that tunnel and coming out on the other side, by making that journey, that I gained so much. Today I feel lucky. I am grateful for the lessons I have learned and for the treasures I have found in my challenges. I have learned that it is important to choose carefully the company you keep. I have learned the importance of having compassion for others. I have learned that it is during tough times that we discover what we're capable of. And I have learned that none of the trappings that we all run after—success, career, money, fame—really feed our soul. They don't come close.

People who meet me today remark on what a great life I have. And I do! I'm in good health. I have a wonderful relationship with my daughter and son-in-law and two fabulous grandchildren. I'm close with my parents and my family. I have a lot of friends—good friends that I can count on. I've written two books and have an active and rewarding professional life. And every day I thank God for what I have, because fifteen years ago it was a very different story. That's why I constantly remind myself that I can never take my life and my happiness for granted. Not one of us can. And that's true at any age.

I try to live the concepts in this book every day, because I now know that I am the architect of my own life. If I want to continue to have a good and happy life, there are things that I need to do, every day, to make that happen. And what I need to do now in my fifties is different from what I needed to do in my twenties or thirties.

We're all going to have setbacks, problems, and challenges. Let's be honest; all of us do. But it's *how* we meet our challenges that determines our lives—especially now. This is the age we start to care, really care, about whether our lives have deeper meaning than we've known. Whatever our personal circumstances, life is not the same at midlife as it was in our youth. We view things differently. We can focus better. We can choose. And while we might not ask for *more*, we do ask for *true*. How wonderful that can be.

My story might sound atypical, but in reality, every one of our lives is unique. What is reassuring is that we all have common threads, challenges that we share. My wish is that the Ageless Living Principles will help you understand that you can be happy, healthy, and beautiful. You can appreciate who you are and live a life that's sound and true. You can be spiritually grounded, and connected to friends and family, and enjoy what life has to offer at midlife—and beyond.

Warm wishes

Doris

Our deepest fear is not that we are inadequate.

Our deepest fear is that we are powerful beyond measure.

It is our light, not our darkness, that most frightens us.

We ask ourselves, who am I to be brilliant, gorgeous,

    talented and fabulous?

Actually, who are you *not* to be?

You are a child of God

Your playing small doesn't serve the world.

There's nothing enlightened about shrinking so that

    other people won't feel insecure around you.

We were born to make manifest the glory of

    God that is within us.

It's not just in some of us; it's in everyone.

And as we let our own light shine, we unconsciously

    give other people permission to do the same.

As we are liberated from our own fear, our presence

    automatically liberates others.

—Marianne Williamson, *A Return to Love*

The Adventure

I wish I could promise you that your life is about to change. But that is for you to determine. The truth is that it takes a lot more than just a set of rules or advice about living to experience the adventure that is your true life: it takes effort, it takes the will to change, and it takes love. What I can promise is that with a sincere and open heart, anything you will for yourself is possible.

The reality is that your life can change *if* you make certain choices and do what is within your power to put them into action. The principles in this book will give you the tools to create a life that is full and true, the life you *know* you were meant to live. But you and only you can make that happen.

marvelous midlife

As women at midlife, we can finally take a deep breath and exhale. We have arrived at the gateway, that marvelous middle place where we are perfectly positioned, poised between where we have been and where we are going. We can look back from this unique vantage point and draw wisdom from all the experiences we've had; and we can also look forward, ahead of us, to the many exciting years to come. At this wonderful time in our lives we each have the power to choose what the years ahead will look like. Midlife presents us with so many diverging paths, so many opportunities, that these years are potentially the richest of our lives.

The best parts of our lives come together at midlife. We have health, energy, experience, and perspective. We have the vitality of our thirties and the wisdom of all our years. We have a large capacity to love and understand, and we have the compassion to live life more fully than we did when we were younger. Midlife can bring a generous sense of humor and a wonderful sense of proportion—who among us can't laugh more easily at what once might have brought us to our knees?—and it can deliver from friends and family the love and support we need to carry us forward. The framework of our life is set. Now, more than at any other period of our lives, we are in a position to make the most of what we have, to decide the course ahead.

> *Life is either a great adventure or it is nothing at all.*
> —HELEN KELLER

live true

Midlife is the time when we begin to ask the important questions: How can I make my life more meaningful? What should I be doing now? What am I meant to do? If my children have grown and left home, what is my role now? Do I still have the same value? How do I manage to deal with the changes in my body and in my life, and still keep a positive self-image as I get older? Is it all downhill from here? The questions we ask ourselves can really be distilled down to this: "Am I living the best life I can? Am I living true?"

How do we live our true life? What would it look like? Is it even possible to have a "true life" with all the day-to-day pressures we face? Well, it is possible. In fact, it has never been more possible. We are at the best time of our lives. Right here. Right now. It is up to us to determine what today will bring, and what the coming years will look like. Life at midlife is filled with transitions and challenges. There are so many ways we can go. That's why it is so important to experience these years with a true and open heart.

True life is lived when tiny changes occur.

—LEO TOLSTOY

We've never been in a better place, or at a better time, to choose for ourselves. We've never been in a better place to make positive changes in our lives. We've never been in a better place to use the wisdom we have gained over the years, and to make the choices that will allow us to live our true life. Yet, at midlife, some of us may feel defeated by our daily routine. We may have given up. We may not have the energy or the courage to venture into new areas. We may have *under*-aimed because we felt *over*whelmed. And because it was easier, we may even have settled.

Everyone has compromised at one point or another. But settling—whether it's with our relationships, our looks, our body, or our dreams—makes us feel defeated, dispirited, and worse, resigned. When we resign we miss out on living our own greatness. We give ourselves up to the needs of others and we take their truth for our own. Resignation is our death knell, whether we are thirty or eighty.

Don't resign. Resist the voice that has made you give up any part of your life, the voice that justifies the uncomfortable compromises, the one that says examining your life is too difficult, or that you're too old to try to get closer to the life you want to live. And about that life you want to live? Well, it's up to you . . .

the age quake

We are privileged to be at a different point in our lives than the generations that came before us. We have the opportunity to see ourselves differently from the way our parents or grandparents saw themselves when they were our age. We know we are not quite the same as we were in our twenties, but for the most part, we are healthy, intellectually active, interested, and have a sense of adventure and spirit much younger than generations before us.

Midlife is almost the beginning of a second life. As baby-boomer women we are creating this defining moment in time when we, together, can transform the concept of the aging process. We are the first generation of women to want something more from getting older, something more than has been shown to us. We may have grown up on attitudes and images that have placed women our age in the background, but we're certainly not about to be put in the background ourselves.

We are in the midst of what I call The Age Quake. Consider it. Some sixty million women in the United States are over the age of forty. Sixty million vital, powerful women who have helped shape the last thirty years—and more—are now over the age of forty. And we are a force to be reckoned with. We've been elected to office and we've flown into space. We've been appointed to the Supreme Court and we've broken down barriers. We've raised children and we've raised hell. We are not going to contribute to our decline by letting our health and our looks go. We are not going to fade away.

Life shrinks or expands in proportion to one's courage.

—Anaïs Nin

When I was told by the beauty and fashion industry that I was over-the-hill and no longer had a place in it—at thirty-eight!—I thought to myself, "Something is very wrong here." I felt very strongly that I was at a time in my life when I had something I could really offer. I believed that my age was an asset—not, as they emphatically insisted, a liability. It had taken me that long to find my own strength and to develop a personal viewpoint that was meaningful to me. If the industry was saying that I no longer had any value, then it was also saying the same thing about all women my age. This thought moved me to action. I had been inside the beauty business for more than twenty years. I knew I was in a position to change their thinking.

I headed to the libraries. I pored over research, read every article I could, and finally put together the evidence that supported my conviction. I discovered I was part of a wave of baby boomers, one-third of the population. Imagine that—forty-three million women strong! Yet, my industry, the beauty industry, wasn't addressing us at all. In fact, we were being dismissed. Products meant for women at midlife were being shown on twenty-year-old girls. There were no images of us. We were invisible.

That is a very loud message. Whether we perceive it or not, that message says: "You who are in your forties, you who are at the prime of your life, you who have the economic power to buy our products . . . you are not relevant. You must be camouflaged, represented by a different image. A younger one. You as you are have no value." Whether this message is picked up consciously or subconsciously, it goes very deep, working on us in a devastating way. We buy the message as we buy the product. We end up actually believing the negative implication that we, at midlife, are somehow not acceptable, that we don't have value. We have been traded in for a younger model. Literally.

True beauty evolves with age.

I had a different vision of beauty, an idea that true beauty is something that evolves as we do. True beauty has to change at each age. We never stop being beautiful. Our beauty is just different. True beauty is intelligent, a beauty to live with and grow with. And it is that difference we have to discover.

Armed with this realization, I began to knock on doors with a new message, trying to get the beauty industry to see the truth that women everywhere have known for years: true beauty includes a woman's inner life and develops as she does. After many knocks on closed doors I found that my idea of true beauty was slowly being accepted. At first, only the women within the beauty industry shared my vision and what it could mean. Remember, this was still a male-dominated industry. Then, slowly, the doors finally opened and I found myself in the position of spokesperson for my generation. And I was passionate about it.

CNN brought me on to discuss the changing role of women in the industry. Estée Lauder used me as the face and spokesperson to launch a new product designed for women in their forties, to an overwhelmingly positive response. I was surprised and moved that, after all this time, women still remembered me and were interested in my message—although, when I thought about it, we really had grown up together. I received a great many letters from women who had reached midlife along with me, seeing my photos in the magazines over the years. They knew I was a single working mom and that seemed to comfort and reassure them. I was thrilled by their words of encouragement, how they felt inspired by finally seeing a fellow forty-year-old in the pages of the magazines, talking at health conferences, delivering a message that was not solely about beauty products but about health and happiness too.

I then started a wonderful collaboration with L'Oréal. Right away, the people at L'Oréal understood and supported my idea that not only did women—*all* women—need great products, they also needed information about how they could live fuller lives. At the very beginning I presented to them what I thought women today wanted out of their lives, what was truly important in their busy schedules: more value, more information, more support. At every level everyone at L'Oréal "got it!" With great enthusiasm, the company threw its energy behind my ideas of supporting women and worked hard so that those ideas reached women everywhere. By backing my efforts at lectures, talks, and women's conferences, to making ovarian cancer its number one women's cause, the company really demonstrated it cared. And I am grateful.

I have worked with L'Oréal for ten years now, and I'm a regular contributor to *The Early Show* on CBS, bringing reports on beauty, health, and well-being to women of all ages. It has been fifteen years since the beauty industry told me I was over-the-hill and would never work again. So, who says there isn't life after thirty-five?

claim your life

We usually know how to start out in life. Our first choices are clearly marked out for us: we go to school, attend college (if we are fortunate), apply for jobs, build a career. We may fall in love, marry, have children, and raise a family. But, after we hit these benchmarks, the path becomes less clear. The choices grow more confusing. What happens next? What do we strive for now? Where do we go from here?

At midlife, we may be wondering for the first time in our lives, "What am I *meant* to do?" The kinds of things that have driven us before may not motivate us now. We may no longer have the desire to reach certain goals—to own a bigger house or make more and more money. We may, however, want more meaning in the things we already have: our relationships, our work, our family, ourselves.

At midlife, we need to understand that we may be going through more inner and outer changes—and *bigger* changes—than at any other stage of our life. We may see certain events or circumstances as no longer important or relevant. We may be reassessing our career, evolving our responsibility as parents, modifying our role in our extended families, and perhaps most importantly, adjusting our self-image. As we reach midlife, many of us feel motivated to reassess what we had set out as our life's goals, and what we have accomplished up to now. And we may want to make some adjustments.

My effervescent friend Mary Lou Quinlan had reached the pinnacle of success in her field—CEO of a large advertising agency in New York City. Much lauded and honored, she was, she says, "where *everyone* wanted me to be!" Mary Lou had it all on the outside, but she wasn't happy. The passion that drove her success had faded and it was beginning to affect her, both physically and mentally. She

> *You need to claim the events of your life to make yourself yours.*
>
> —ANNE WILSON SCHAEF

had few resources left. Prudently, instead of continuing until she burned out, she made a brave decision and asked for five weeks off to "find herself" again.

During that time, Mary Lou says, she became completely selfish: "I did something that is very difficult for a woman to do. I did *whatever* I wanted and never asked myself, 'What do I *need* to do?' " She calls that period "my bratty weeks." She spent time with her family and friends. She did "frivolous and happy things!" She took classes she had always dreamed of taking: kick boxing, ice skating, salsa, and meringue. She started a journal to connect to her spiritual side. She "de-cafed" and went on a protein diet. She read books she had always wanted to read. And all during her time off, Mary Lou compiled a list of things she loved to do that made her happy and excited, things that were the opposite of being a CEO. At the end of her "walk-about" she looked at her list and discovered that not *one* of the things that she did at work was on it. So, against everyone's advice, she decided to quit her job and do what she was truly passionate about: start her own business advising companies about the real needs of women. Five years later, Mary Lou's company, Just Ask a Woman, is a very successful consulting and concept development company. Now a role model for other women in business to follow their potential, their passion, and their dreams, Mary Lou says that she is "healthy, happy, proud, and creative." She had the insight to listen to her inner voice and the courage to follow it.

Having the courage to make the most of your life can begin at any age, but it's important to realize that the sooner you make up your mind to take action, the faster you will see results. Why wait a moment longer to find out what you are capable of? And why settle on very modest expectations for your life ahead? You only need to want to do your best and have the discipline to carry it out, and that is true for all of us no matter what our age or circumstances.

We learn to do something by doing it. There is no other way.

—JOHN HOLT

My son-in-law, Christian, has worked as an actor since the age of nine. I admire him because he is always working toward being the best person he can be. Instead of complaining that he missed out on certain "normal" childhood things, he decided to do something about it. At age thirty-one, he sat down and made a list of all the things he wished he had done, and committed himself to doing them. In other words, he consciously chose to live his unrealized life.

One of the first items on Christian's list was to get his high school diploma. He bought all the books he needed, found a tutor, and began to study day and night. After all these years, he finally got his GED—while in his thirties! When the exam results came in the mail, Christian left me a wonderful phone message saying, "I just wanted you to know, since you were so excited for me: *I DID IT!*" He then went on to the next item on his list, earning his black belt in karate. After six months, he got his purple belt—halfway to his goal. And he is going down the list, marking off one item after the other, breathing life into each of the "unlived" parts of his life.

the power of potential

Today, more than ever, we have the inner resources to live our true lives. All we need is know-how: the tools to get there and the energy to use them. But, because we *do* need energy to enter new territory, energy we may not feel if we are unsure of the road ahead, we can become resigned to a small life rather than take chances. When we live our life on a small scale, less than what it could be, there is no new blood to carry us forward, no new energy to help us change, evolve, and grow.

We all have the capacity for development and achievement. That is our potential. Unrealized, that potential becomes an unlived life. When we don't connect with it, when we aren't able to access it, we live below our own promise and end up living a smaller life. We begin to feel a disparity between the life we are living and the life we long for. This can make us feel depressed. And make us very angry. And even make us sick. Because of this disparity, we struggle within, often blaming our discord on something else—circumstances, other people, life, God. Yes, it takes courage to look at your life. It takes bravery to make things happen for yourself, sometimes by yourself. It takes daring to live up to your potential, to breathe life into your unlived parts. But what's the alternative?

There is no agony like bearing an untold story inside you.

—Zora Neale Hurston

Why should we live up to our potential? Why should we develop our true self? Because no one helps the world by being a small person. You help the world, your family, your partner, your friends, your community, *yourself,* by being your biggest, kindest, and most scintillating self. And the fabulous part of being at midlife is that we are able to say, "It's now or never." Now is the time we can create more value, find more meaning in our lives. We may have looked to others at different times in our life to complete us—partners, children, friends, employers—but today, as wise women, we understand that we have the power to complete ourselves.

If you are like me, then somewhere inside there is a tugging feeling, a yearning to be your true self and live your true life. We all feel it, even if we don't quite know what that true self is. Somewhere, deep within us, there is an inner blueprint that longs to be created in the outer world. It's like being turned inside out: We want the person we truly are to be revealed to the world. Inside each one of us lies greatness. We want to access our greatness and offer it to the world. We *want* our own light to shine. We want to make meaning out of the mundane. It is our gift, both to receive and to give.

Life doesn't always turn out as expected. We often start out with open arms, brimming with hopes and dreams, ready to embrace the world, certain that it will be a better place because of our efforts. We soon realize that life has twists and turns awaiting us, and so we try to manage the best we can with the challenges that each one of us must face.

Greatness doesn't have to mean grandness. Our greatness may lie in finding the cure for cancer, or it may lie in showing love to a friend who has cancer.

Today, more than fifteen years have passed since my husband died, that time I now refer to as "the black hole." During those fifteen years, I juggled taking care of my daughter and searching for a way to support the two of us in an industry that revered only youth. I watched people around me move ahead with their lives when I felt mine was standing still. But I had no other choice. I had to move forward. I took stock of where I was and accepted that I had to start over. I shed a few tears, faced some fears, and managed to find my strength—and, thank God, a good dose of humor along the way!

The difficulties that I went through gave me the chance to develop parts of myself that I might never have dared to confront. And although at the time I wished that I had left well enough alone, my journey gave me the understanding that our problems—I prefer to call them *challenges*—are our greatest gifts. Our problems offer us a chance for transformation. They dare us to change our lives.

Today, I realize that because of those challenges I have created a bank of wisdom I draw upon daily. This wisdom, this understanding of life and my role in it, is very precious to me. I now know that true wisdom can't be bought or learned in school, nor can it be taken away. I now know that when we acquire the understanding and wisdom that our experiences can give us, and work to keep a positive attitude, no matter what the obstacle we face, we do grow.

It's been a long journey, and I've learned so much along the way.

I have learned that when we reassess our lives—whether we are forced to or simply choose to—we always receive gifts.

I have learned that it is the journey, not the destination, that holds the greatest insights and rewards.

I have learned that there is a direct connection between a rich inner life and true happiness.

I have learned that our problems are opportunities for transformation.

I have learned that true wisdom is earned over time.

I have learned that we never know what's on the other side of hardship.

And, I have learned that the times we feel most burdened by life's challenges are when we have the *most* possibility.

The Principles

Living true for the rest of our lives, realizing our highest potential at every age—that is how we all want to live. And that is Ageless Living.

Can we really live agelessly, even as the years tick by? Can we really live a life full of energy, vitality, curiosity, promise, fulfillment, and beauty? Yes! Ageless Living means, first and foremost, living unrestricted by an age or by a time. It also means being ready to embrace the true possibilities of our lives. Because when we let go of what restricts us, what makes us small, then we release ourselves from what holds us back from our own infinite possibilities. And when we do, those possibilities can come to life.

Gravity, the aging process, our own thinking, the thinking of others, our losses—all of these elements can bring us down. But we can use the Ageless Living Principles to uplift us, to expand and breathe life into those areas that are most important to our health and well-being, but to which we may not have paid as much attention as we should.

We live agelessly when we free ourselves from our perceived limitations of age, when we can live unrestricted by a date on our driver's license. *This is ageless living.*

We live agelessly when we let go of what holds us back, when we embrace our age completely, unbound by its grip. And when we live our life agelessly, we are free to explore all the possibilities that open up for us as we go forward. *This is ageless living.*

We live agelessly when we realize the promise in the age we are *now,* and when we are open to discover the treasures in every age. *This is ageless living.*

We live agelessly when we have the courage—whether at twenty or eighty—to proclaim, "I am perfect at the age I am now!" And when we do our world expands and our life gets bigger. *This is ageless living.*

We often feel bound by what we think we are: by being a woman, a mother, a daughter, a minority, rich or poor, too skinny or too heavy. We can feel bound by our emotions: fear, anger, love. And we can also feel bound by our own thoughts: "I'm inadequate." "I'm unattractive." "It will never happen for me." "I don't want to change." "I'm comfortable where I am." When we surrender to whatever we think binds us, we automatically contract. We see ourselves as victims. Age can be one of those things. It can make us feel out of step, not just at midlife, but all through our life.

As women, we often feel we are either too young or too old. In our twenties, we're never old enough, and in our forties we're never young enough. We've been acutely aware of our age at every age. Not any more.

The Ageless Living Principles help us live with the infinite possibilities of each age. They help us live consciously and in the present, allowing us to live all of our "unlived parts." Ageless living teaches us to be aware and grateful: grateful for what we have gained over the years, not frightened about what we have lost. Yes, there are natural limitations: the body's aging process, changing relationships, life's circumstances, our own mortality . . . but the Ageless Living Principles can keep us continually expanding and growing. They breathe wisdom into our life; they assist us in identifying the areas that will help us create that bigger life. They support our evolution.

Midlife is a time of transitions, a crossroads. We can take many directions or paths from here. It can be exciting. But sometimes we need help, and that's where the Ageless Living Principles come in. The principles are sensible, generous values that help us to decide our own ways of fulfillment. As we choose between life's many paths like colors from a palette, we can use the Ageless Living Principles to help us make the individual choices that contribute to the shape and shades of our lives. These choices do not have to lead to grand, dramatic changes. Sometimes all we need is to make small shifts in our attitude to see the way forward more clearly.

The Ageless Living Principles show us the choices and paths that lead us to live our true life, our fullest life, and our highest life. They cover five areas of living that, together, help us stay balanced and happy. Each principle develops a specific area, bringing our whole life into poise. All the principles overlap, working together as pillars to support us. And, as we become more aware of one area of our life, we often find we're more interested and open to growth in another. Using the Ageless Living Principles we can find out where to direct our energies and how to get the most out of life. A guide to the infinite possibilities in each of us, these principles help us realize that we don't have to settle.

Using the Ageless Living Principles in my own life, I have the feeling that everything is right. I have a sense of completeness and happiness, a sense of saying, "Yes!" to all of life. I feel I am part of the whole. I am filled with enthusiasm, understanding, balance, joy, and playfulness. I know that I'm using all of myself, *all* my parts—developing them and being able to offer them to others. These principles constantly guide me to the areas that I need to work on. They help me shape my evolution. When I practice the Ageless Living Principles in my life, I have the experience that I am living life, rather than that life is living me.

THE AGELESS LIVING PRINCIPLES

Look Your Best

Present your true self by taking care of the outside

Nurture Your Spirit

Take time for yourself and develop your inner life

Honor Your Body

Create energy and strength for your best health

Discover Your Wisdom

Draw on your experience and know that you are wise

Stay Connected

Reach out to family, friends, and community

Principle One:
Look Your Best

**Present Your True Self
by Taking Care of the Outside**

This is not a "beauty book." Although I certainly have a lifetime of tips to help you look your best, I want to encourage you to believe that true beauty radiates from a deep, inner place. The most important thing to know about beauty is that the old adage is not true: beauty is *not* only skin deep. Beauty is a reflection of all life's moments—joy, sorrow, love—and it begins inside long before it shows itself on the surface. Beauty is found in exuberance, sadness, and peace. Beauty is experience. And beauty at midlife is a ripe, rich treasure. Look Your Best is a very important part of a spiritual look at your true life. That is why it's presented here as the first of the Ageless Living Principles.

This principle does offer some advice on what you can do to look gorgeous on the outside; however, the approach is holistic, involving mind, body, and spirit. For me, midlife beauty is not so much about *tricks of the trade* as it is about harmony—health, energy, enthusiasm, and a strong sense of self. At midlife, beauty and spirituality are connected, reflecting each other in the packaging that is us. We want to look our best, not necessarily out of vanity, but because we want to be proud now of who we have become—and who we are becoming.

respect yourself

When we cherish something, whether it's a new home we're thrilled to have, a car we've saved for, or even a pair of shoes we've had our eye on for ages, we treasure it, we care for it, we treat it with respect. Our home becomes our castle—even if it's only a one-room castle—our car is kept polished and protected from the elements, and those shoes . . . God forbid it might rain the first time we wear them! So why would we treat our personal appearance with any less value or honor? We need a healthy well-cared-for body that represents who we are. We need it to interact with others, to move around with, to love and be loved. Our body *does* serve us well. Think about it. Where would we be without our dear body, no matter what its size or shape? Why shouldn't we take pride in its upkeep and appearance?

Taking the time to care for ourselves by looking our best, we honor our inner life. And when we like who we are we take the time to look our best. My friend Michele has a ritual of always carefully putting on her lipstick before she goes out, as well as right after eating. We often tease her about it. She says, "Putting on my lipstick is part of taking care of myself. It changes my attitude and my state of mind. Applying lipstick honors a sensual side of myself." Breaking into laughter, she admits, "It also controls my eating. The better I look, the less I eat!"

Taking care of ourselves is usually one of the first things we let go when we are depressed. In fact, neglecting our appearance can be one of the first signs of depression. If we don't value ourselves, then of course we are going to think, "Why bother?" A dental hygienist once told me that she can tell which patients are depressed, because they have stopped brushing their teeth. And doctors have told me that patients have improved, almost immediately, by doing something as simple as washing their hair or putting on lipstick. They healed faster, weren't in as much pain, and didn't ask for painkillers as often.

> Two of the saddest words in the English language—*why bother.*

If taking care of ourselves can have such a positive effect on us when we are sick, imagine how it can uplift us on a daily basis. When we make even a small effort to look better, it always makes us feel better. I know of a sleep-deprived new mother who burst into tears the first week at home with her infant daughter. Instead of being worried, her sister kindly teased, "I know you're going to be okay. You're wearing ear-rings!" Tears turned to laughter.

After years of working with women, friends, and family, through lectures, workshops, and informal sessions, I have seen how confidence builds when people are shown how to make the most of their unique appearance. They gain freedom and empowerment when they see the results—no matter what their age or gender. My father, who has just turned eighty, is a man who truly belies his age. He is curious about seeing and doing everything that is new, and he surprises people who are much younger with his ability to keep up. He is a great example of ageless living and a wonderful inspiration for me.

> *The beautiful rests on the foundations of the necessary.*
> —RALPH WALDO EMERSON

Having gone through the Depression, my dad is very careful of waste. And that awareness extends to his clothing. He feels he should wear his garments until they wear out. No matter what my mother has suggested about updating his wardrobe, he has steadfastly resisted. Well, on a recent trip to Italy, I decided to take up my mom's case and see what I could do by offering to treat my dad to a new set of clothes. At first he hesitated, but maybe the Italian version of *joie de vivre* took hold, because he generously allowed me to have my way. So we went to town. Literally!

My father is already a handsome man, but in his new simple yet classic wardrobe, he was transformed. Out went his usual drab, plaid shirt and in came a soft coral cotton pullover and a navy cashmere sweater that highlighted his thick, white hair. He was, in a word, gorgeous. As the compliments showered over my father everywhere we went, I saw his posture become straighter, his step lighter. These new clothes had taken years off his age. By hiding in outfits that were out of date, he had become invisible. After years of working hard and supporting a family, my dad kind of forgot about himself. But the simple act of wearing new clothes that complemented him, and receiving the attention that he did, brought him renewed life. I felt privileged to remind him that he deserves to look his best. And, that's pretty darn good.

your best you

I believe that deep down we all want to look—and be—our best, no matter how busy or stressful our lives. At a recent health conference in San Diego I gave a talk to women on using the Ageless Living Principles. Before the conference I was fortunate to be able to work with a group of volunteers who had agreed to use the principles as a guide to help transform their lives. The women were either in the military or were married to someone in the service. One woman was a helicopter pilot, another was a drill sergeant, and a third was a military wife with the full-time job of raising three young children. All were bright, attractive women excited to be getting together for self-improvement. This wonderful multiracial group had one thing in common: they wanted a transformation on a deeper level, something that would change them, that would go deeper than just cosmetics, something that they could continue to use in their lives.

We gathered around the table as each woman shared what she secretly wanted most from the session. One woman wanted to feel more confident when she entered a room. Another wanted to be able to take care of herself *in very little time* as she had small children to run after. And yet another laughingly begged, "*Please,* help me do *something* with my hair." In a matter of minutes, amid much laughter, we became a positive, supportive group of "girlfriends." All women at midlife with a lot of responsibility resting on them, they were not obsessed by their appearance; nevertheless, each of them wanted tools to help her look her best, a little extra know-how to gain a new self-assurance and freedom.

Together, we pinpointed the things they most wanted to change. We cut, styled, and colored their hair, and I showed them how to apply their makeup so they could do it quickly and easily themselves. It might have been an outer change, but as these women developed a part of themselves they had previously neglected, an inner transformation took place too. These small changes helped them blossom, giving the women self-confidence and a whole new sense of self.

We honor our life by presenting our true self to the world, by keeping ourselves cleaned, groomed, and well dressed—even if only in a simple pair of jeans. Showing respect for ourselves, we show respect for life. When we complete daily beauty rituals such as washing our hair, keeping our nails clean, bathing or showering, we are more ready to face the day and all its challenges. Why wouldn't we want to be dressed in clothes that are clean and presentable? Or keep our skin glowing with health, protected from the elements with moisturizer and sunblock? These are simple, basic ways we can all look our best.

> Looking your best is looking like you feel good—and *feeling* like you look good.

Feeling that we look our best gives us the courage to dare. And looking our best gives us an opportunity to renew our confidence. When we feel good about ourselves—when we believe in ourselves—we want to participate in life. We feel strong and self-assured, and that self-assurance lets us focus our attention freely on the present, instead of being distracted by a constant stream of worries scurrying across our mind, convincing us we are less than perfect.

When we don't feel good about ourselves we tend to focus on our imperfections, or on what is less than important, like that piece of double-edged tape we've used to fix our hem. How many of us have worried about how we look before we go out to a party or a job interview, or if what we're wearing is right for the occasion? And who hasn't, at some point, had a bad hair day? When we wear clothes that don't fit or don't feel good, when we don't make an effort with our appearance, we can feel distracted and vulnerable. No matter who we are, negative thoughts about our appearance can cause us moments of anxiety, and sometimes hours of insecurity, all adding up to lost time. Focusing on what we consider to be our shortcomings—fretting about our appearance—we feel insecure and less able to engage with others. We miss out on the freedom of the moment because we are not present. Lacking confidence in how we look, we don't feel free to fully participate in the world around us, to enjoy ourselves or contribute to the enjoyment of others. We lose opportunities. We feel diminished.

> *The real sin against life is to abuse and destroy beauty, even one's own—even more, one's own, for that has been put in our care and we are responsible for its well-being.*
>
> —KATHERINE ANNE PORTER

Self-care is not the same as vanity, and paying attention to our appearance doesn't make us superficial. Looking our best reflects how we feel about ourself. And it's not just surface. Women sometimes have the misconception that if we do focus on our looks, we're not something else. If we are pretty, we are probably not smart. If we spend time primping on the outside, we must have nothing inside.

A psychotherapist that I was "making over" was anxious I might make her look so pretty that her patients wouldn't take her seriously. Here was an accomplished professional woman who was frightened to let her beauty shine through because she thought it would detract from her intelligence and professionalism. What a shame. She needed to realize that her beauty was just as much a part of her as her intellect and her insight. She needed to accept that her beauty *belonged* to her.

We all need to embrace the truth that looking our best—taking care of ourselves—is part of a whole that resonates positively to the outer world. More importantly, it resonates positively to the spiritual beings that we are.

love the one you're with

It's important that we recognize how good we look now. My friend Barbara recently said to me, "I looked at pictures of myself from ten years ago. I wish I'd known at the time how good I looked." She is in her fifties, and as I looked at her beautiful face, I said, "You can know that now."

We have no idea how we look in action, how we look when we're connecting with other people, how we are when we're laughing, what we radiate when we're passionate about an idea, or in the throes of love. It is within our joy, our inner light, that our beauty lies. We have no idea of the beauty that always radiates from us. I find that many women, like Barbara, are ten years—or more— behind their own beauty. When we look back at ourselves years later with that much more wisdom and experience behind us, we finally see it. We look at old photos and think, "Why didn't I know how good I looked?" Why do we have to miss it? Imagine if we could know it now. Imagine the freedom we would gain by letting go.

> *Beauty is not caused.*
> *It is.*
>
> —EMILY DICKINSON

Open yourself up to the possibility that you too may be like Barbara. You may not see your own beauty today. You may not have a button nose or shell ears, but you are beautiful. Why not realize it today? Why wait another ten years to enjoy it? As I told Barbara, "You look good now!"

When you know you are beautiful, you can let go. When you unhook your attention from your looks, you are free to grow. Until that happens, the nagging voices of doubt pull you away from the truth of your own beauty.

It is our birthright to be beautiful, and it is our responsibility to cherish the beauty of each age. As women at midlife at the beginning of this new century we have the right—here and now—to say, "I look good," without feeling that we have to tack on that dreadful little phrase, "for my age . . ." Now is the time to accept and define our own beauty, value, and worth. Cosmetics may give us a lift, but if we aren't able to leave our house in the morning comfortable in our skin—*bien dans sa peau*, as the French say—there isn't a cream in the world that's going to make us feel better. A new eye shadow may add a sparkle to our lid, but it won't put a twinkle in our eye; only our own positive attitude will give us that.

Why is taking care of our appearance an important part of being the best we can be at midlife? Because beauty is as much about how we see our life as it is how we look throughout our life. To me, looking our best says, "I like the age I am now. And I like the age I am becoming!" Our appearance is the first thing others see when they meet us, the first thing they see before they get to know the wonderful person inside. Offering our true self to the world says, "I like who I am. I am alive. I am ready to participate."

Sometimes, by midlife, we are so used to giving to others that we forget to give to ourselves. We may feel we shouldn't spend time or money on our looks, or we may think, "What's the difference, I can't turn the clock back anyway." We may find the vast array of beauty products bewildering and not know where to begin. Or, we may simply be uninformed, believing that the skin damage that comes from direct sunshine is "nature's way" or that looking our best needs to be complicated, with an expensive array of treatments such as botox injections, chemical peels, and face-lifts. It doesn't have to be that way. In fact, looking good is a lot simpler than we think.

position yourself

The easiest way to improve your appearance is by improving your posture. Simply standing up straight can take a good ten years off your age and five pounds off your body! That's why it's one of my favorite "beauty secrets." But there's more. How you hold yourself actually says a lot about the way you position yourself in the world. Think about it. When you stand up straight, you look and feel assured. Your attitude conveys self-respect, which signals to people that you want them to treat you with respect. When you slouch or wilt, however, you tell people that you're tired and that you don't want to be bothered. And chances are they won't want to be bothered either.

When I went with some friends to watch a tea ceremony being performed, the Zen master called our attention to the importance of sitting tall, saying that good posture was really about our attitude toward life and our respect for self. He told us that when we sit and stand straight we are communicating to our problems that all is well, that we are in control. It changes the way we see the world and the way we feel about ourselves.

Never bend your head. Always hold it high. Look the world straight in the eye.

—HELEN KELLER

Good posture is something we need to pay special attention to at midlife. As our body ages, as gravity beckons us to "come on down," we find ourselves fighting against the pull of the natural aging process. Nature seems to want to contract our bones and change our self-image—all those things that can shrink us—but there is something we can do about it.

An approach such as the Alexander Technique can help us adjust our posture to relieve the stress and tensed muscles that can cause misalignment. The Alexander Technique teaches us different ways of moving—and *thinking* about moving—so that standing straight takes less energy than slouching. It makes us think about conserving energy and relaxing in everything we do, and it teaches us how to release unwanted muscular tension. Think of it as a blueprint of what good posture should look like, be like, and feel like.

Proponents of the Alexander Technique believe that proper balance and alignment of the body, what some people refer to as "muscular attitude," is essential to good health. I know that I've found this method of holding my body helps me to resist stress and move with ease.

There's no reason we have to surrender to the visual of the older, bowed, sinking, resigned woman. The weight of our head, our breasts, and the force of gravity may pull us forward, out of alignment, but we can counteract this by strengthening our back muscles and standing tall. I've noticed that when my back muscles don't have enough strength, even just standing still takes effort. I tire easily and feel pain in my lower back. But, when I stand with proud, straight posture, I feel strong. And that's when I convey vitality, strength, and optimism to the world.

posture perfect

- Check out your posture in a mirror. Are you slouching? Is your head down or your back bent? Try to stand so that your ears, shoulders, hips, knees, and ankles make one straight line. And relax. Straight doesn't mean stiff.
- Stand against a wall. Is there a large space between your lower back and the wall? If so, use your tummy muscles to try to press your lower back into the wall,

pulling in and pulling up. This will give you an idea of how you can feel when you lengthen and properly position your spine.

- Pulling in your tummy keeps your posture straight. So, when you're sitting, concentrate on pulling your belly button toward your spine. (I often do this in my car.)

- Check your posture the old-fashioned way, by balancing a book on your head. Practice so that you can take at least ten paces before the book falls off.

- Put Post-its on your computer or around your work space reminding you to "Stand up straight!" or "Sit tall!"

- Engage in exercises such as walking, running, yoga, and Pilates. They help strengthen and tone stomach and back muscles.

- Stress can be a posture killer. It can make you look as if you're carrying the weight of the world on your shoulders. Finding ways to deal with stress will almost naturally perk up your posture.

- When sitting, try to use a firm chair with a high back. Put your hips far back against the chair, and make sure your knees are at hip level or lower. Avoid hunching forward when you're working or driving.

- Heavy breasts can cause you to slump, so exercise to strengthen your back muscles and make sure you have the proper bra support.
- Make sure you have a healthy diet full of calcium to ensure the health and strength of your spine.

keep moving to look your best

Exercising sends oxygen and nutrients to our skin, giving us a natural, healthy glow. An activity as simple as walking can relieve stress, burn calories, and promote energy—all of which help make us look great. In fact, a recent study at the Royal Edinburgh Hospital in Scotland found that exercise can make us look and feel up to eight years younger! They found that the equivalent of three brisk one-mile walks a week make us look that much younger while improving our circulation, bone strength, and our immune system. "It's not all in the genes," they say. The ravages of time can be reversed. According to the study, the key is activity, both intellectual and physical, *and* a good sex life!

As we get older, our metabolism slows down, and we begin to notice our bodies changing. I remember my friend's surprise while contemplating her slightly drooping tummy in the mirror, just after her forty-second birthday, and her wry lament, "Oh, now I see why it's called *middle* age."

Looking your best means helping your body, through exercise, *be* its best. And no matter what shape you are in, you can make a difference with only a little effort on your part. You can start by having a great walkout. It's easy *and* fun. A good walk should take at least thirty minutes. Spend the first five minutes walking at a normal speed, increase your stride and pace for the next twenty minutes, then slow down for the last five. (If you're feeling energetic, you can increase your walk to forty-five minutes.) When walking, pay particular attention to your posture—shoulders back, stomach in. Breathe deeply. Remember, fresh air feeds your skin.

Exercise. You don't have time not to.

If you exercise in the morning, have a piece of fruit or an egg before you start out. Leave time for digestion. If you exercise after work, make sure you've had enough lunch. You need to be nourished to exercise effectively and you need to refuel after exercise too. Trainers tell me to eat at least twenty minutes after working out. I always carry a snack with me. Sometimes I'll take dried fruit or a handful of raw almonds. Other times I'll treat myself to an energy bar, like Luna bars for women. They're great in a pinch. (My favorites are Lemon Zest and Nutz Over Chocolate. For a special treat I reach for Chocolate Peppermint Stick—Yum!)

the stress connection

Everything we do affects the way we look: the foods we eat (or don't eat), the products we use, how we feel about ourselves, our work, our finances, our relationships. They can all add up to stress. Stress is a response to a demand. It's that simple. Whether the demand is placed on our body, our mind, or our emotions, the resulting stress can make our heart beat faster and make us sweat more. It can leave our mouth dry and our hands cold. It can change our appetite and disturb our sleep patterns. Stress can also manifest itself with aggravating skin problems like acne, hives, eczema, canker sores, and rosacea, by weight gain or loss, or by the physical effects of sleeplessness.

Stress releases adrenaline, that old *fight or flight* response, which in turn can affect the facial muscles, making your face appear tense and older.

There are many solutions that help me combat tension: walking, being in nature, taking time out with my friends, being with my grandchildren, writing in my journal, exercising, reading, cooking, gardening, and doing anything creative. The list is endless. Whatever unhooks us from the daily grind and nurtures our spirit will help cushion us against stress, and a big payoff is that it will do wonders for how we look.

Pampering ourselves is one way to relieve stress—it's good for our looks, as well as our spirits. We can relieve stress with something as simple as a manicure or a pedicure. Giving ourselves the luxury of a massage or even a regular hair appointment can do us a world of good. My mother has a standing weekly date at her favorite hair salon that she has kept, rain or shine, for years. She calls it her "Saturday morning pickup." My mom says she looks forward to Saturday all week because this time she takes for herself both relaxes her and gives her a little bit of luxury after working all week.

I meditate regularly. But when I feel stressed, when my thoughts and emotions overwhelm me, I particularly appreciate the benefits that meditation brings me. Meditation connects me to a deep reservoir of calm and quiet. It helps me view the challenges of the day from a better place. Meditation also quickly leads my body to a more relaxed state, reversing the effects of stress on my appearance.

I cannot say enough about the tremendous benefits we get from deep breathing, especially when it comes to stress. When we're tense, we are almost cut off from our breath, which is our life source. That's why *pranayama* breathing in yoga is so valuable. We learn a deeper breathing from the lower abdomen that brings us calm almost immediately and helps everything in the body circulate, which all shows up on our skin.

Shallow breathing also reduces our energy, making us feel fatigued. When we do take time to pause and focus on our breath, taking long, deep breaths, in and out (at least three), we can both see and feel the effects—in the lightness of our step, in our sense of rejuvenation, in our skin's radiance. You don't have to make any special effort to take a good, long, deep breath. You don't have to put on a leotard and sit cross-legged. You don't even have to leave home. You can breathe deeply anywhere at any time, standing or sitting. Just do it—any effort is better than nothing. The best way, though, is to breathe through the nose, filling the lower lungs and exhaling slowly back out through the nose.

Taking long, deep breaths whenever we can remind ourselves is another of my instant "beauty secrets."

You feel calmer when you breathe deeply, and you look better. Breathe, breathe, breathe—even if you have to put Post-its near your phone, on your computer, or over your kitchen sink to remind yourself!

it all begins with skin

Beautiful skin is possible at any age, and with just a little bit of care we can all have clear, vibrant skin that radiates vitality and health all our life. We usually know when we're neglecting our skin. We may think we're too busy, or we don't know how to make ourselves look better, so we end up doing little or nothing. And, over time, little or nothing becomes a lifestyle. To look our best, we need a sensible approach to the basics. And we need to be consistent.

I've always taken good care of my skin, but today I'm even more disciplined in its daily care and protection. I need to look my best in the least amount of time, so I have my routine down to the basics: cleanse, nourish, protect. And I'm faithful to it. It's important to have a good, basic skin-care routine. Only when we know what works for our skin on a daily basis—when we're in balance—can we know what to do when changes occur. And changes will occur. Constantly. After all, our skin is regularly exposed to the elements—wind, air, smoke, pollution, and that dreadful offender, the sun. Gravity too has its effects (no matter how hard we work to fight it) and our skin also reacts and responds to such things as changes in season, hormones, diet, and medication.

So how do we cope with these changes? Is there anything we can do to slow them down? I believe it's important to relax about the natural aging process. We all will show some signs of aging: a few wrinkles, expression lines, a softening in tone, a change in texture. It's important to accept these changes, to regard them as evidence of a full life, as outward indications of life happening. But only up to a point! Part of being wise women may be accepting the natural aging process with grace, but that doesn't mean we can't do something about it. We can take steps to change what is in our power to change, and to protect our skin from further damage in the years ahead. The good news is that we can stave off unnecessary damage to our skin and keep a vibrant appearance. All it takes to keep our skin looking its best is to learn about the aging process, and how to prevent the most damage.

a change of habit

Many of us have read about certain causes of cell damage that affect the way our skin looks and feels. We may recognize the terms *free-radical damage,* but do we know what it means? Free-radical damage happens throughout our life, but the effects really start to show in our thirties as our skin's production of collagen and elastin, the "scaffolding" that holds it together, naturally declines. To make it very simple, a free radical is a cell that is missing an electron, or part of itself. These free radicals are present everywhere in our daily environment, especially in the air. They steal what they need from our healthy cells, causing our skin to break down. When a healthy cell is robbed, it too becomes a thief to complete itself, and before we know it, we have a lot of little burglars, pickpocketing our youth.

The effects make themselves known as wrinkles and sagging skin before our time. That's why, when it comes to caring for our skin, I believe that the best defense is a good offense. And one of the best ways we can help our skin prepare for that offense is with good habits. There is simply no such thing as clear, vibrant skin—skin that radiates vitality—without a healthy lifestyle. Our skin registers damage before any other part of our body when we don't treat it well. It records stress, lack of sleep, pollution, and bad habits such as using alcohol and cigarettes. There are many ways we can work toward having great skin: by being physically active (which increases circulation and reduces stress), eating nourishing whole foods, drinking enough water, protecting skin from environmental damage (especially the sun), and choosing products that best suit our needs. At midlife, the most important thing we can do is to not give up. Our goal is terrific skin at every age, for the rest of our life. And the only way to achieve that goal is to reexamine our habits, good and bad.

A balanced diet is more than a healthy way of living, it's a beauty secret. Many skin problems, like dull skin, uneven texture, acne, dry lips, and split nails, can mean a vitamin deficiency. Though many skin-care products now have vitamins, they aren't concentrated enough to make a real difference in our overall health. (In fact, sometimes our skin-care products may mask problems that would be better treated by a balanced, nutritious diet.) One of the best ways to have really good skin is to make sure that we get enough vitamins from the inside out. Just think of it as eating well to have great skin!

- *Alcohol* can affect our skin, leading to broken blood vessels and spider veins, especially on the areas around the nose and mouth. Alcohol can also produce facial flushing and trigger rosacea.

Excess alcohol (more than one drink a day) prevents the body from absorbing the necessary nutrients and vitamins that our skin needs. It can also dehydrate us—that's why we end up with hangovers. (What counts as a drink? Five ounces of wine [a small wineglass], 12 ounces of regular beer [a mug], 1.5 ounces of liquor [scotch, vodka, etc.])

- *Caffeine* dehydrates the body, and when we are dehydrated our skin just doesn't have the resiliency it should. Drinking an excess of coffee, tea, and sodas that contain caffeine can actually drain the body of water, causing our skin to sag and look wrinkled. (Caffeine also elevates blood pressure and makes our heart work much harder.)

- *Deep Breathing* gives us so many benefits, from relieving stress to bringing much-needed oxygen to our brain, our blood, our cells, and all our organs, including our skin. When stress hits, many of us literally hold our breath. Our breathing becomes shallow, which can speed up the aging process, affecting our memory and concentration, and making our skin look dull.

- *Nutritious Foods* are a must for great skin. Good food provides the nutrients necessary for the production of the collagen and elastin that support our skin's structure and make it look young and firm. A diet lacking in protein will affect the quality of our skin, hair, and nails as our body shuts down to preserve the protein it needs. Vitamin A—found in carrots, broccoli, and sweet potatoes—helps us create new skin cells. Vitamin C from citrus fruits, red peppers, and berries is essential in cell formation. And vitamin E, found in dark, leafy veggies, as well as nuts, seeds, and flaxseed oil, retards aging and may even prevent age spots. Getting the best nutrition possible allows our skin to help protect against environmental assaults—sun, wind, radiation, and the sea of bacteria in which we all function—and it also helps us optimize the healing of any wounds. Remember: You are what you eat!

- *Overwashing* is definitely drying to the skin. It can irritate, inflame rosacea, and cause what's called irritant acne. Overcleansing with detergent soaps can remove the top protective layer of oils and leave our skin vulnerable to the drying effects of the environment. There is a misconception that repeated washing of oily skin or acne will help it improve. Yes, you want to keep your face clean, but bear in mind that over-washing may actually make acne worse.

■ *Sleep* deprivation affects our hormones, which disturbs our energy level, mood, appetite, sexual interest, and the quality of our skin. Lack of sleep can also trigger release of the hormone corti-sol—our stress hormone. Overproduction of cortisol *ages* our skin, giving us a drawn, sallow look. Lack of sleep can also affect how much or how little water we retain, which can cause a change in skin tone.

Your sleeping position can not only worsen wrinkles you may already have, but sleeping face-down or on your side can actually create new wrinkles and creases on your face. The best sleeping position is on your back!

■ *Smoking* causes serious damage to our bodies and is a major threat to healthy skin. Smoking actually breaks down cell walls, making skin wrinkle, droop, and sag. It also robs skin of oxygen, produces free radicals, and—as if that weren't enough—is one of the leading causes of premature aging, along with sun damage. Smoking inhibits blood from nourishing our skin, aging it much more quickly, and it also contributes to poor circulation, making it harder to heal from surgery. (But you don't need me to tell you to quit . . .)

- *Stress* affects our thyroid and cortisol levels, causing mood swings, erratic appetite, and loss of energy. It can also trigger troublesome skin conditions such as acne, rosacea, psoriasis, and dandruff. Stress can cause a swing in hormone levels, which may result in a decrease in sleep, or erratic sleep. And that can show up on our skin as loss of elasticity, dryness, and breakouts. Be conscious of stress levels in your life. Don't forget to breathe!

- *Sun* is the single most damaging factor to our skin, so staying out of the sun is the best possible way to safeguard our complexion. It's important to understand that not only sun *burning*, but sun *tanning* represents damage to our skin. The best defense is year-round UVA/UVB sun protection of *at least* 30. And remember, sun damage is cumulative over our lifetime.

- *Water* needs to be consumed throughout the day. It keeps the body hydrated—providing more energy—and it gives skin a healthy glow by helping to flush away toxins. Our skin contains molecules that bind water together and plump up the skin. If our skin is hydrated it will remain firm. If it is dehydrated it will stay "tented" when we pinch it. Dehydrated skin loses resiliency and will become wrinkled. And because we lose water constantly, even through an action as simple as breathing, we need to replenish our water intake by drinking enough all during the day. Don't wait to feel thirsty before you take a drink, and bear in mind that seltzer, juice, and even soup can count toward your daily quota.

what's your type?

Our skin is held together by a sophisticated support structure of collagen and elastin. As we grow older, that support structure doesn't renew itself as it once did, meaning that our skin loses its ability to spring back into place. That's the phenomenon that occurs when we release our smile, only to realize that little smile lines stay where they were. As we age, our body's natural oil production slows and our skin becomes thinner and drier. Our skin may need even more moisture as we approach menopause because a decrease in estrogen slows oil production even further. Those of us who have struggled with blemishes in our thirties and forties can rejoice, however; that extra oil in our skin will give us some additional defense against fine lines and wrinkles. Unfortunately for many others, acne can also be accompanied by dry skin, making it difficult to determine their skin type. And make no mistake about it. You can't care for your skin properly unless you know what type of skin you have.

We might not have the same skin type we had a few years ago. We might not have the same skin type we had even a few months ago. But it's important to know our current skin type if we are to care for it the best we can. Consider the women who think they have dry skin when in fact they really have skin that is damaged, either from the sun, the environment, or alcohol. They use a moisturizer for dry skin, but instead of improving, their skin just gets worse.

How do you determine your skin type? If your face gets shiny an hour after you wash it, then you have oily skin. If your skin feels dry and tight throughout the day, then you have dry skin. Most of us have combination skin: oiliest through the center of our face (the T-Zone, where most of the oil glands are), and drier toward the sides.

The most foolproof way to determine your skin type is to see a dermatologist. A dermatologist can be your skin's best friend, in good times and bad. He or she can help you with something as simple as keeping your skin healthy and looking its best, to performing more aggressive procedures such as surgery. A dermatologist can help you find a great program suited to your skin type, one that takes into consideration your ethnicity, your environmental conditions, and your daily schedule. Of course a dermatologist can also offer advice on medical procedures such as skin peels, laser, or botox.

As well as being able to diagnose and treat all skin, hair, and nail conditions (and help you find the right treatment for problems from rough flaky skin to persistent acne), a dermatologist will be able to tell you what type of skin condition you actually have. Many of us, for example, think that we have acne, when in fact we may have one of the "acne imposters" such as epidermal cysts or rosacea. Self-treatment for the wrong condition can be harmful (and expensive!), so if you're concerned about your skin, take the time to visit a dermatologist and make sure that your skin-care efforts are not being wasted.

Think of your dermatologist as an educator, a qualified professional who can advise you on changes in your skin due to hormones and the natural aging process. Dermatologists can provide guidance on the sea of products available out there on the shelves. They can separate fact from fiction about the latest treatments and techniques, and can also advise you about what's going on in product R&D (research and development). Some dermatologists, such as Katie Rodan and Kathy Fields, even formulate their own products. Drs. Rodan and Fields created Proactiv Solution (see Resource Guide), which a great many people swear by for the treatment of acne and uneven skin tone.

When it comes to choosing a dermatologist, do your homework. Most are caring, respectful professionals. Nevertheless, I've heard a few unfortunate stories of dermatologists dismissing women with "What do you expect for your age." Thankfully, these stories are rare. Nevertheless, I suggest you consult the American Academy of Dermatology (see Resource Guide) and try to get referrals from friends and colleagues. Read what you can. Take your time and shop around. Choose from one of the many dermatologists who have compassion for their patients and their concerns, one who is receptive to answering a question as simple as "What night cream should I use?"

> After forty, you should visit a dermatologist and be checked annually or biannually for skin cancer, one of the easier cancers to detect and prevent.

This is a good time to grow old. With all the technology available, with all the R&D going on, we have the ability to give our skin the best care available. And yet many women still hesitate before seeking professional advice. According to dermatologist Dr. Lydia Evans, many women in their forties and fifties are interested in seeking a dermatologist for help in "aging gracefully," but often feel guilty about asking for the extra attention. "I find it generational," says Dr. Evans.

"My younger patients are open to taking care of themselves, but *our* generation has tremendous guilt. Like their moms, they think they should just put some cold cream on their face and leave it at that." *Don't* just leave it at that. *Do* take the time to care for your skin. Know what your skin needs. Know how to protect it. Consult a dermatologist and find out what works best for you. Great skin is easier than you think.

beauty bottle basics

No matter what brand of skin care you use or whether you buy your products at the department store or the drugstore, you should know what's in the bottle and what's likely to work for you.

INGREDIENT	SKIN TYPES	BENEFITS
Alpha-Hydroxy Acids (AHAs)	Dry, damaged, lackluster skin; fine lines and wrinkles	AHAs come from fruits, sugarcane, and milk. AHAs speed cell turnover, revealing the healthy, smooth skin underneath. They protect skin against surface wrinkles, and may work to repair some environmental damage.

INGREDIENT	SKIN TYPES	BENEFITS
Retinol and Vitamin A	Damaged skin, acne-prone skin, uneven skin tone, lack of firmness or elasticity	Retinol, a form of vitamin A, helps to speed cell turnover and increase collagen production. Also used to reduce pigmented spots on the skin.
Vitamin C	Fine expression lines and wrinkles, damaged skin, lack of firmness or elasticity	Works to reduce the appearance of fine lines and wrinkles. Protects against UV damage, and evens skin tone. Also increases collagen and elastin.
Vitamin E	Fine lines and wrinkles; oily, blemished skin	An antioxidant, used as a treatment for acne. Protects against UV damage and helps to minimize expression lines and wrinkles.
Collagen	Dry, damaged skin with fine lines and wrinkles	As we get older, collagen production slows, which can lead to sagging skin. Collagen (a protein) helps to plump up and firm the skin.
Hyaluronic Acid	Dry, aging, or damaged skin; oily skin that is dehydrated	Hyaluronic acid traps moisture within the cells of the skin.

INGREDIENT	SKIN TYPES	BENEFITS
Coenzyme Q-10	Dry, damaged, and lackluster skin; fine lines and wrinkles	Coenzyme Q-10 lives in every cell of the body and is an antioxidant that works to slow free radical damage.
Emu Oil	Dry skin; oily skin that is dehydrated	Emu oil seems to have fewer of the side effects of other moisturizers, such as clogged pores, but is more emollient than mineral oil (an ingredient used in many "dry skin" products).
Shea Butter	Dry, dehydrated skin; skin that suffers from rough patches	Shea butter, a fat extracted from the seeds of the shea tree, is used to soften skin and hair, and prevent dryness.
Tea Tree Oil	Combination or oily skin	An antiseptic and natural cleanser, tea tree oil soothes skin irritation and blemishes. Also speeds healing.

the rule of three

Most women are as familiar with the notion of a three-step
daily skin-care routine as they are with the habit of brushing
and flossing. You probably know these steps as cleanse, tone,

and moisturize, but I've altered them slightly so that you can be sure to protect your skin as well as moisturize it. Let's take a look:

1 Cleanse and tone

2 Nourish

3 Protect

COMMON-SENSE CLEANSING AND TONING

Basic Cleansing The first step in rejuvenating our skin is a gentle and thorough cleansing, twice a day. You may want to use a different cleanser in the morning than in the evening, or you may want to use a refreshing toner—or even a splash of water—to help you feel early morning fresh. It's vital, however, to thoroughly cleanse our skin at night before bed. Remember when we were younger, stayed out late, and jumped into bed with all our makeup still on? Of course we wouldn't do that now. . . .

Be sure to *always* wash your hands before cleaning or moisturizing your face. Bacteria can easily be transferred from fingers to products . . . and onto your skin.

We all know it's a must to cleanse our skin, but sometimes we do cheat. We fall into bed after a long day, telling ourselves that one night of mascara won't matter. But it's important to wash away the day's grime every night so that

SOAP OPERA

I shudder when women tell me they use regular soap on their face, the same soap they use on their body. Soaps can often be too drying for aging and sensitive skin; they strip it of its natural oils.

As we age, our skin isn't able to replace these oils as quickly as it did when we were younger. Still, that squeaky-clean feeling can be enticing. So, if you do like using soap, try one made for sensitive skin, such as Neutrogena's Extra Gentle Cleansing Bar.

The most gentle and effective way to cleanse is to use a creamy cleanser first, to get the makeup off, then follow with a gentle *face* soap to remove the residue.

not only do we clean away makeup and debris that clog our pores, we also remove dead skin to reveal the healthy new skin underneath. Cleansing helps prepare our skin to be nourished, and it also helps to wash away the day's stresses. I love to use my cleansing time to unwind, contemplating the events of the day before snuggling into bed.

- Choose creamy, liquid cleansers that won't strip the skin of natural oils.

- Look for plant-based products; they're milder than animal-based.

- Select fragrance- and detergent-free soaps, especially if your skin is sensitive or dry.

- Use mild or lukewarm water to rinse. It helps dissolve soap more effectively than cold water.

- Don't use hot water. It strips the natural oils, can aggravate sensitive skin and rosacea, and can cause broken blood vessels by increasing the blood flow to the surface.

- Use small, round facial sponges to cleanse. I like the drugstore sponges called UpStage. These great little cleansing sponges (they cost about $1.30 for a small bag), soften up nicely when wet, and make marvelous mini-exfoliators that help remove aging skin cells.

- Pat the skin dry with a clean, soft towel. Don't rub. That will pull the skin. Pay special attention to the delicate areas around the eyes—no pulling or rubbing.

Basic Toning Toners prep our skin for moisturizers and makeup, making them easier to apply. I like to use them after cleansing—I love the refreshing feeling that they give me—especially during the hot summer months. Midlife skin is fragile, so make sure to use the appropriate cleanser morning and night, then use a gentle toner, followed by a cool splash of water. Because our skin becomes drier at midlife, it's important to look for toners that are alcohol-free, or formulated for sensitive skin. This is true, even if you have the oiliest skin. (For problem oily skin, try a prescription-strength Retin-A cream.)

- Look for ingredients such as rose water, or purchase a 100 percent rose water from your local health food store.
- Choose natural plant extracts like cucumber, aloe, and chamomile—all gentle on your skin.
- Be careful of toners with isopropyl alcohol if your skin is sensitive or dry. It can aggravate your skin, and many toners do contain it. Remember to read the labels!
- The old tried-and-true witch hazel, often used as an astringent, is alcohol-based and much too drying for most skin. I would avoid it.

Supplemental Cleansing A mild cleansing exfoliant once a week helps moisturizer penetrate your skin. It also slows down the aging process by eliminating the top layers of dead skin that get "glued" in place by air pollutants, cosmetics, medications, oils, and heat. You may be surprised to find, when you gently exfoliate, how baby-soft and wrinkle-free the layers underneath are.

There are two popular and effective kinds of exfoliants: manual scrubs and moisturizing formulas. The manual scrubs, made up of tiny grains, actually scrub the dead cells off the skin's surface. But you must be gentle, because they can tear your skin. Use small circles and apply light pressure. Never pull or tug the delicate skin on your face. Many moisturizing formulas that contain alpha-hydroxy acids (AHAs) and retinoids (products that contain derivatives of vitamin A) come from fruit, sugarcane, or milk, and work on your skin to remove that top layer of dead skin cells over a period of time. Bear in mind that AHAs may be a better choice if your skin is too sensitive for retinoids.

how to pick an exfoliant:

AHAs and Retinoids

- Start with the mildest formula, such as a 4 percent solution of AHA.
- Begin using the product every other day. If your skin is doing well after two weeks, continue on a daily basis. If you notice redness, try it only once a week or try a retinoid product, such as retinol or Retin-A.

- Be fanatical about wearing an SPF—either in a sun-block or a daily moisturizer. AHAs and retinoids cause the skin to become more sensitive to the sun.

Scrubs and Grains

- Choose a product with tiny round grains, in a moisturizing cleanser or cream, or just use a fluffy face cloth.
- Avoid using "scratching scrubs" with large uneven grains. They can make little tears in the facial skin.
- Exfoliate in the shower, when your skin is still wet.
- Use tiny, circular motions and *very little* pressure.
- Never exfoliate the delicate skin under or around the eye.
- If you use a facial brush, first test the softness of the bristles on the back of your hand. Make sure they give easily under pressure.

NECESSARY NOURISHING

Basic Moisturizing   At midlife, we need to keep moisturizing our skin, inside and out, summer and winter. Moisturizers not only make the skin feel better once you apply them, they also help to "trap" moisture and create a protective layer against environmental damage.

If it's hot and humid, oil-free moisturizers such as L'Oréal FUTUR.e Moisturizer for normal to oily skin or Crème de la Mer's oil-free moisturizer deliver a shot of cool hydration. If the weather is dry and cold, thicker creams such as L'Oréal Paris Age Perfect Day Cream or Lancôme Primordial Intense provide more emollients to create a barrier to protect skin from damaging elements.

There is a difference between daytime and nighttime moisturizers. At night, our skin's cell turnover speeds up and creams are more quickly absorbed. So take advantage of this antiaging secret by using a good cream specially formulated for nighttime such as Estée Lauder's Advanced Night Repair, or L'Oréal's Age Perfect Night Cream. Maybe that's why they call it our "beauty sleep!"

"All-natural" skin-care products with plant-based ingredients lose their effectiveness quickly because they don't contain preservatives. It's best to toss any skin products after six months, whether they are all-natural or not. Toners and alcohol-based products can last up to one year. I like to write the date on my products when I buy them.

NOURISHING BASICS

	WHAT TYPE OF SKIN DO I HAVE?	WHAT SHOULD I LOOK FOR?	WHAT CAN I USE?
Normal Skin	Not excessively oily or dry. Weather changes mostly don't affect your skin.	Any creams or milky lotions that are lighter, to maintain moisture level as is.	Eucerin Protective Moisture Lotion SPF 25 Clé de Peau Beauté Emulsion Protectrice Tendre L'Oréal Paris Age Perfect Day Cream Topix Replenix Green Tea Cream
Dry	Flaky, easily irritated. Especially dry and flaky in winter.	Thicker creams that are water based (instead of alcohol) and are more moisturizing. Creams with hyluronic acids, which hold moisture. Choose products without fragrance or essential oils that can be drying.	L'Oréal Paris Age Perfect Day Cream Estée Lauder Daywear Protective Anti-Oxidant Crème Clinique Moisture On-Call Orlane B21 Crème Fluidratante Catrix 5 Correction Cream

	WHAT TYPE OF SKIN DO I HAVE?	WHAT SHOULD I LOOK FOR?	WHAT CAN I USE?
Oily Skin	Shiny look. Need to wipe away oil. More greasy in hot weather. Trust your fingers.	Use the lightest formulations. Choose oil-free, gel formulas, or serums that are lighter and disappear more quickly than creams. Facial scrubs and toners can be used more frequently. Use a night formula that contains retinol, a form of vitamin A.	Shiseido Pureness Matifying Moisturizer Oil-Free Kiehl's Sodium PCA Oil-Free Moisturizer Lancôme Hydra Contrôle Mat La Roche-Posay Effidrate
Combination Skin	T-Zone is oily and the outsides are normal to dry.	Use an oil-control toner or pad to wipe the T-Zone regularly and a moisturizer for normal or dry skin along the sides.	L'Oréal Paris FUTUR.e Moisturizer Normal to Oily Shiseido Pureness Moisturizing Gel-Cream Neutrogena Maximum Strength Oil-Controlling Cleansing Pads La Roche-Posay Toleriane Soothing Protective Light Facial Fluid

	WHAT TYPE OF SKIN DO I HAVE?	WHAT SHOULD I LOOK FOR?	WHAT CAN I USE?
Sensitive Skin	Can be any type: sensitive and oily or sensitive and dry. Reacts easily to different chemicals.	Go by your skin type first. Use lotions and creams. Look for little to no preservatives, fragrance-free, no detergents. Be careful of alpha-hydroxy, or chemicals.	Neutrogena Moisture for Sensitive Skin Oil of Olay Sensitive Skin Active Hydrating Fluid Crème de la Mer Moisturizing Lotion La Roche-Posay Toleriane line of products
Problem Skin— Acne	Breakouts. Blackheads and whiteheads.	Use non-comedogenic, oil-free products and creams that won't block pores. Look for beta hydroxy/ alpha hydroxy washes. Use cleansers with facial scrubs. If you are not allergic, use sulphur-based creams or masks.	L'Oréal Paris Pure Zone Skin Relief Oil-Free Moisturizer Aveeno Clear Complexion Daily Moisturizer Lancôme Acne Côntrole Daily Acne Medication Gel-Cream

	WHAT TYPE OF SKIN DO I HAVE?	WHAT SHOULD I LOOK FOR?	WHAT CAN I USE?
Problem Skin— Damaged	Brown marks, wrinkled, usually dry. Your skin may have been exposed to sun and now has lost the ability to keep in moisture. May also be windburned or overexposed to the cold.	Moisturizing creams. Use antioxidants, which remove fine lines. A bleaching agent to lighten brown spots. Retin-A and glycolic acids.	Lancôme Vitabolic products and Re-Surface products L'Oréal Paris Revitalift Shiseido Future Solution Total Revitalizing Cream Lustra by Medicis Tri-Luma
Problem Skin— Dehydrated	*See* Dry Skin	*See* Dry Skin	*See* Dry Skin
Problem Skin— Rosacea	Your skin appears sunburned, flushed, or blotchy pink. Aggravated by heat and cold. Tends to flush with hot drinks, alcohol, spicy foods.	Stay away from chemicals unless prescribed by a dermatologist. Shark cartilage is soothing, decreases blood vessels. If not allergic, products that are sulphur based can be soothing.	Clé de Peau Beauté Essence Appaisante Joey New York Calm & Correct Gentle Soothing Moisturizer Catrix Rosacea Therapy GlyTone Sulphur Masque

supplemental nourishing

- Apply a moisturizing mask once a week, such as Lancôme Hydra-Intense Masque or Clé de Peau Beauté Masque Transparence.

- No matter what your skin type, switch to milder skin-care products; they are gentler to aging skin.

- Look for words such as *moisturizing, gentle, for sensitive skin, nourishing,* or *replenishing* on product labels.

- Vitamin C is a great antioxidant. The jury's still out, but it may even have a stimulating effect on collagen, making your skin look and feel firmer—and younger. (It's hard to keep vitamin C stable, though, so look for products from established companies. Try Lancôme Vitabolic or La Roche-Posay Active C.)

- Avoid fragrance in products if you have allergies or sensitive skin. Read labels if you have known allergies.

- Switch to creamier moisturizers with aloe vera or hyaluronic acids to create a protective barrier from the elements.

- Be cautious when mixing creams. For example, creams with copper peptides are very popular now, but if applied next to a product containing vitamin C, both solutions will lose their potency.

- Keep a purse-size water sprayer with you and spritz your face (and the surrounding air) throughout the day.

- Buy a humidifier to "moisturize" your home and office, especially in cold weather when indoor heating can rob your skin of moisture. At around thirty dollars, it's a great investment in your skin. (Be sure to change the water every day so that bacteria doesn't form.)

POSITIVE PROTECTION

Basic Sun Protection   My number one beauty secret is sunblock, sunblock, sunblock! Every day, rain or shine, winter or summer. Wearing sunblock has become second nature to me. I keep it in my purse, my office drawer, the car. And I constantly remind women to apply it to those places we don't often think of: the back of our hands, our neck, our chest, and especially the back of our legs, where we get the most sun exposure. Even though most of us know how important wearing a high enough SPF is to our health and our skin, I still have trouble getting people to remember to put on sunblock—and to apply enough of it. Most women mistakenly believe it isn't necessary to wear sunscreen *every* day, year-round. But it is, even in winter or on a cloudy day.

Anyone who knows me knows to what lengths I will go to protect myself from the sun. I always wear an SPF of 30 or above, I often pull my long sleeves over my hands if the sun is glaring, and I'm regularly protected under hats and sunglasses. I will cross the busy streets of Manhattan just so that I can walk in the shade, and on occasion I've even been known to resort to gloves and an umbrella!

A tan may look good for the moment, but it's actually evidence of injury to the skin. And when the tan fades that damage remains and eventually shows itself as premature aging of our skin—or worse, skin cancer. If we know that skin cancer is one of the more preventable types of cancer, why would we choose not to completely protect ourselves?

We must realize that a year's worth of incidental sun exposure— walking outside to the car, to get the mail, to chat with a friend—all adds up to the same skin damage as a week spent baking on the beach without sunscreen.

As my daughter, Ryan, was growing up I struggled to get her to wear sunblock. It's only now, at age thirty, after a few years of living in the California sun, that she's beginning to see the damage it can do to her skin. For a long time, she had difficulty finding the right sunblock because she doesn't like a greasy feeling or any scent. Now, finally, she's discovered a light, scent-free and oil-free sunblock that works for her body, Natura Bissé, and she loves Crème de la Mer sunblock for her face. You can always find the right sunblock for you; the important thing is to wear it.

In choosing the right sunblock, try to pick one made by a company that knows skin care, one supported by years of research. I love Neutrogena's waterproof SPF 45 sunblock. Sea & Ski makes a good affordable block with zinc and an SPF of 50. There's a brand in France that I

Remember to be generous when applying sunblock. It's better to use too much than too little.

find fantastic called La Roche-Posay Anthélios. It's creamy and moisturizing, not greasy. You can get it from most dermatologists. Also, Shiseido makes a great face sunblock, and I love the tiny Mustela sunsticks for babies, which I throw in my purse. (See Resource Guide.)

Sun Protection Basics

HOW OFTEN: Every two or three hours—more often, if you're in the water or perspiring.

HOW MUCH: Use an amount equivalent to a shot glass, which should cover the face, neck, and hands.

WHEN: Apply at least thirty minutes before going into the sun.

TYPE	HOW IT PROTECTS	ACTIVE INGREDIENT	WHO SHOULD USE IT	PRODUCTS	ADVANTAGES
Chemical Sunblock	Protects by absorbing sun's rays and causing them to change on the skin.	Parsol 1789	Good for those whose skin is less sensitive—some skin breaks out with chemicals.	Neutrogena UVA/UVB Sunblock 45	Blends in with the skin; more aesthetically pleasing; absorbed instead of "sitting on top" of skin.
Physical Sunblock	Blocks rays physically from reaching and harming skin.	Zinc and/or titanium dioxide	People with light-sensitive or very fair skin.	La Roche-Posay Anthélios 60 Mustela Total Sun Protection Stick	Best blockout; less skin irritations so more people can wear it.

- Look for a sunblock with both UVA and UVB protection, or "broad-spectrum." UVA, the "aging" rays, lead to wrinkles and premature aging; UVB, the "burning" rays, cause sunburn and skin cancer.
- Check the ingredient list on your sunblock. If it doesn't contain either zinc oxide or Parsol 1789 (also called Ivo Benzone), then it will not protect you properly.
- Use an SPF of at least 30 or above.
- Colored sunblock has the bonus of showing you the areas you may have missed.
- Don't use last summer's sunblock—it's no longer effective. Sunblock has a shelf life of about six to eight months once opened.

which sunblock is right for you?

Gels—Dry more quickly, better for oily skin, don't stain clothes.

Creams and lotions—Provide more moisture, better for mature and/or dry skin.

Foundations with SPF—Make sure they have broad-spectrum UVA and UVB protection; if not, use *over* your sunblock. Apply throughout the day, especially around the eye area.

Increase your sun protection—wear sunglasses, hats, and
protective clothing. Glasses for ten dollars with UVA
and UVB protection will be as effective as a pair for
one hundred dollars.

Wash your summer clothes in Rit Sun Guard Laundry
Treatment. It gives an SPF of 30, protecting you from
the burning rays that seep through your clothing. It
lasts up to twenty washes.

hair apparent

How do we keep our hair looking great throughout our years?
By keeping it clean, conditioned, and well trimmed. It takes
very little time and attention to care for our hair properly, and
great hair can help us look good and feel confident. Hair that
isn't well cared for—hair that is greasy and limp, damaged, or
badly colored—says that we just don't care. And why would
we want to communicate that?

The first rule of hair care is to keep it clean. I know it
seems obvious, but when life is hectic and things get stressed,
sometimes the most obvious things get missed. Not doing
your hair in the morning may shave ten minutes off your
schedule, but if those ten minutes get carried throughout the

day as insecurity about your looks or fussing about your hair, then you haven't saved anything at all.

Make sure to use a shampoo formulated for your hair type and routine. If you wash your hair every day, use a very mild shampoo such as Neutrogena Clean Replenishing or L'Oréal Paris VIVE Fresh-Shine. I also like Philip B. Peppermint and Avocado shampoo, especially when I'm slow to get started in the morning—it's like a peppy wake-up call for my hair! If you color your hair, be careful to use a product formulated to protect the color, like L'Oréal Paris Color VIVE or Neutrogena Clean Color-Defending shampoo. Look for products that are easy on the hair and watch how your hair reacts to them. The weather, your general health, and your stress level all affect the condition of your hair, so it's likely that you'll need to try changing formulations from time to time.

As we get older we usually need to put more moisture back into our hair. The products we use, the medicines we take, our hormones, the weather, constant coloring, or just the continual use of hot hair dryers and clips and rollers can all cause our hair to become damaged and dried out. That's when it's time for some tender loving care. Use a conditioner *every* time you wash your hair. If your hair is fine or you feel that conditioner weighs down your style, apply conditioner only to the ends, making sure to avoid the roots.

I make sure to use a conditioner each time I wash my hair. I reach for a heavier one during the summer months when my hair gets dried out from chlorine, the sun, or the sea. I've tried many different products, but I've discovered one that has made a big difference in my hair, making it shinier and more manageable; the whole line of Kérastase products. For my hair, which is curly and can be dry, I especially love Kérastase Oleo-Relax, which is deeply hydrating, and Lumi-Extract cream, which I smooth on my hair and leave in. The trick is to rub a little back and forth in your hand, warming it, then lightly stroke over flyaways or through dry hair. You can find the Kérastase products in most specialty hair salons (see Resource Guide).

Whether you have long hair or short, make sure to have it trimmed regularly. A trim will keep the dead ends at bay and will also ensure that your hairstyle has movement. A little trim can make a big difference. My sister Dari has always had a beautiful mane of waist-length copper brown hair. It's her trademark. Each time I see her, I give her a cut and help color and condition her hair. Recently, I gave her a quick trim and deep-conditioned the length of her hair, and the results were amazing. Both her daughters, Zephora, who is thirty, and Quinlyn, who is only fourteen, couldn't stop admiring their mom. With only a subtle hair trim and a hydrating conditioning, Dari looked years younger!

If you want to change your look, change your hairstyle. Changing your hair, whether with a new color or the latest cut, is the most immediate and effective way to make a difference in your appearance. It's also the fastest way to give yourself a lift. It's always so much fun to see. Carol Hamilton, President and General Manager of L'Oréal Paris, is known for her chameleon style. I never know who she is going to be next. "My personal style starts with change," Carol says. "And so does my hair color. Every month! I've been every red, from copper to burgundy, and every shade of blond, from honey to highlights." And Carol looks great in all of them. "Changing my hair color keeps my attitude confident."

We change our hair to feel good—and look our best—but at midlife and beyond we also need to change the way we care for our hair. As our hair grays, the texture becomes drier and wirier. And during menopause, one in three women experiences some hair loss. Now is the time we may dare, maybe for the first time, to think about "dramatic" hair changes, as well as to consider new ways to care for our hair. As Carol says, "It's the ultimate way to transform your look and keep your style vibrant and interesting."

what color?

Looking your best means finding the color and cut that is best for you, one that flatters the shape of your face and the color of your skin, and that you can easily maintain. And, if you decide not to color, which can also be fabulous, then make sure your gray is a happy and healthy gray. Pay attention to the cut and use special products to take care of your beautiful gray hair. My mother has the most lovely white hair: snow white, not yellow, not blue. I'm always admiring it. It's a

> You can tell that a new color doesn't work with your skin tone if you have to wear more makeup to match your new hair color.

very "young" white, a happy white, and it frames her face with a luminous light! Top colorist Louis Licari recommends that women with gray hair try rinses that will minimize the yellow cast that gray hair sometimes takes on. There are also silver "toners" (which are actually light blue) that you can use. But if you decide to go with a silver toner leave it on for only half the time. You don't want to look like a blue-haired little old lady!

I've seen women who color their hair and look fantastic, and women who are salt-and-pepper—or completely white—and look equally amazing. Whichever way you choose, just make sure that your cut and color suit your face, your personality, and your lifestyle. No matter what you do, just make sure that you have the time and resources for the upkeep of your hair. There is nothing more aging than unkempt, uncared-for hair, white roots showing, orange or otherwise badly colored hair, or even purple hair—which can sometimes happen with white hair.

One thing you should know is that as we get older our skin color changes; it looks thinner, more translucent, and at times takes on a yellow cast. So, we have to pay attention to complementing and flattering our skin with the right hair color. The color that suited you in your twenties might not be the right one for you in your forties or fifties. I had hair that was blue-black when I was younger; that color would be much too harsh for me today.

I suggest making an appointment with the best professional hairdresser you can find, and let him or her guide you. The top colorists I've talked with say to color the hair "band" around the face a shade or two lighter than the rest of your hair; that way, your hair color blends into your skin subtly, looking more natural than a harsh block of color that stops abruptly at the hairline and definitely looks dyed. Steer clear of extreme hair color changes. Darker hair can look monochromatic and drab if you go too far. If you've made a mistake and colored your hair too dark, a professional can "lift" the color and correct it by pulling a lightener through the tiny strands of hair that frame your face.

If you don't want to go for an allover change, highlights around the face can also be effective to brighten your look. Keep in mind that highlights should enhance your look, not change it. Sometimes women get so many layers of highlights that they change their color altogether, making it too light and unflattering. The right hair color should be one shade lighter than your natural color, two shades lighter at most. As Louis Licari reminds us, "Lighter doesn't have to mean blond." If a new shade is too light for your skin tone it will drain the color from your complexion just as gray hair can. Go for "warm" shades, like honeys, golds, caramels, champagnes, or ambers. Avoid "ash" shades, which can make hair appear smoky or drab.

Some women wouldn't dare color their hair at home, while others wouldn't dream of doing it any other way. I visited top New York hairstylist Garren at Henri Bendel's, who admired the color of my hair. I surprised him by telling him it was out of the box: L'Oréal Paris ColorSpa Moisture Actif—Cocoa, my favorite! At-home hair color works for me. I do it as often as I can, because there is less fuss, and I have more control. I do a lot of my own coloring with ColorSpa. At $7.99 in the drugstore, the secret's out.

If you are coloring your own hair for the first time, know that there are two kinds of color: permanent and semi-permanent. Permanents are a commitment—the color can't be washed out. They contain peroxide and ammonia, which lightens your own natural hair color. These products work well for women who are more than 50 percent gray. You will need to touch up your roots every few weeks.

Semipermanents, like the one that I use, last up to twenty-eight shampoos. (The products that contain ammonia last longest.) They can be gentler on the hair, and the color is more subtle. Most of today's semipermanents will not lighten the hair at all. Semipermanent colors blend away gray, and because they fade gradually, less upkeep is needed.

key color tips:

- Don't shampoo your hair just before coloring. It will remove the natural oils that protect the scalp.
- Always do a strand test before coloring all your hair. Color one lock to make sure the shade suits you.
- Deep-condition your hair a few days before coloring. The shade and shine will last longer.
- Protect your hair color from the sun's damaging rays; it will change the tone. Hats or scarves work well, as

do hair "sunblocks" such as Phytoplage or Kérastase Solaire Voile Protecteur.

- Select shampoos for color-treated hair; they're gentler.

- Try a "color depositing" shampoo, like Aveda's, to keep your color refreshed. It contains vegetable color, so it cleans and deposits color, instead of stripping it.

- Swimmers need to know that chlorine and salt can change hair color. Take preventative action with protective products such as Kérastase Bain Après-Soleil Shampoo and Huile Protective.

hair loss

There's a difference between hair loss and thinning hair, both of which can happen as we get older. Even though we may panic when we notice a lot of hair in our brush, rest assured—we naturally lose about one hundred strands a day. The aging process will cause an additional bit of hair loss; if, however, you notice a sudden dramatic difference, like hair falling out in clumps, it's important to see a doctor. Hair loss can be caused by thyroid disease, heredity, hormonal imbalances, a reaction to medication, and sometimes, stress. Thinning hair can be caused by stress, aging, and menopause, and can often be helped with improved nutrition.

If you have thinning hair and want it to appear thicker, try volumizing products such as Privé Amplifying Shampoo or Kérastase Volumactive. They can make individual strands stand apart, giving the illusion that the hair is thicker than it actually is. One dermatologist I spoke with who specializes in thinning hair suggests that dandruff shampoos can also help because they stimulate the scalp, increasing circulation. I would also suggest massaging the scalp with your fingers. It helps circulation, *and* it feels good too. If your hair is fine or thin, avoid heavy moisturizing products. They tend to make thin hair look flat and a little slick or greasy.

Hair saving or restoration products, such as Rogaine, offer even more improvement for women than for men. The company has a line of shampoos and conditioners, Progaine, which are formulated especially for women. The line contains a "thickening" shampoo that works by cleaning and nourishing the hair with a weightless formula. Hair thickening products can provide a temporary "fix," coating each strand between shampoos and making the hair look thicker. Try other hair thickening products from Phytocyane and Nexxus.

the look-your-best checklist

Our mind and body know when they are loved and cared for. When we take the time to do both, we see it immediately in our attitude toward life, as well as in how we look. At midlife, we as wise women know that to look our best is to announce our proudest inner selves. So don't underestimate the power of the connection between how we look and how we feel. Looking our best gives us the energy to tackle change in our own lives, as well as the lives of others. When we look our best, we feel we can take on the world—or at least the day.

- Take at least ten minutes a day to care for your skin by moisturizing and cleansing from head to toe.
- Exfoliate once a week, or when needed.
- Wear UVA/UVB sunblock of at least 30 SPF, always—summer and winter, day in, day out.
- Organize and clean out your beauty products every six months; most have expired by then. Write the date of purchase on each new product, so you know when to toss them.
- Buy inexpensive little plastic baskets from the drugstore—I do. Separate your products by categories:

body, face, cleansers, hair products, and one little basket for extras.

- Healthy hair starts with a good trim. Phone for an initial appointment and schedule your next two appointments in advance. If your roots are showing, or you haven't completely decided to go gray, ask for a color consultation (no commitment required).

- Be sure you eat a balanced diet, full of foods rich in antioxidants.

- Keep healthy foods at home; no junk. If you don't have it, you won't eat it!

- Exercise three times a week for at least thirty minutes.

- Spend one lunch hour this week walking outdoors. But don't skip lunch. Invite a friend to join you.

- When your day-to-day life overwhelms you, choose one meditative pursuit that will calm you. It can be as simple as a warm twenty-minute bath, a five-minute breathing session, or burning essential oils in your room.

- Get at least eight hours of sleep a night.

- Instead of watching television before bed, listen to classical music, read a book, or write in your journal.

- Stay hydrated. Keep water with you at all times.

- Make a conscious effort to replace old negative "tapes" in your head with new positive ones: "I feel great," "I am healthy," "I look my best."

- Post these statements wherever you will see them— on your bathroom mirror, by the telephone, in the kitchen, in your date book, or on your computer.

- Believe in your own beauty.

Principle Two:
Nurture Your Spirit

**Take Time for Yourself
and Develop Your Inner Life**

As we reach our forties and fifties, some of us may feel we need an anchor, a higher sense of purpose. Personally, I cannot imagine life without a spiritual awareness, without an inner connection or an understanding that I am part of a bigger picture. It's important for me to understand that what I think and do, how I treat people, affects me and the world I live in. My sense of spirituality grounds me, allowing me to put my life into perspective. I know I am supported by a spiritual life I can draw upon, not only in moments of difficulty, but during good times as well. For me, spirituality involves a sense of communion with *all* things: nature, mankind, the world at large.

Why do I feel that having a spiritual life is so important for women at midlife, and that we should do everything we can to nurture one? The answer is simple: our day-to-day lives are so often centered on problem solving that we are in danger of losing ourselves in the details. We are occupied with things like getting a report in on time, driving our children from one activity to another, fretting about bills that need to be paid, worrying about our children's passage through their teen years, our job security, the health of our loved ones, our aging parents, retirement planning—the whole range of life's concerns. A single day can involve an endless series of problems and decisions. When that happens day after day and our life becomes relentlessly problem-oriented, demanding a response to one crisis after another, we are in danger of disconnecting from the inner joy that is in all of us.

Don't get me wrong. Solving problems is normal. It's something we all have to do. But without a sense of higher purpose those problems can get us down.

And where do we end up in the process? If the answer is "last on the list," then we are missing out—missing out both on what is, and what could be. When we confuse *doing* with *being* we lose the chance to experience the nurturing that comes from living our true life, and living it joyously. But when we find ways to nurture our spirit, we fill ourselves back up with the joy we need to enhance life's pleasures and tackle life's challenges. We allow ourselves to live true.

Don't lose the possibilities to the problems.

Contemplating a spiritual life can be uncomfortable if we've lost touch with the intangibles or don't feel a connection with God and all living things. Life is a miracle, and we need to always remind ourselves of that, in both good times and bad. Sometimes, however, we forget that we are all part of a bigger picture, and when that happens we run the risk of missing the vastness of life, of becoming cut off from the nourishment that a strong spiritual life provides. If it were up to me, I'd have us all put down "Nurture My Spirit" *first* on our daily to-do list.

By developing ourselves with spiritual practices that take us within, we are supported by immense power and deep truths.

To do . . .

1   Nurture my spirit.

2   Share my joy.

3   R-E-S-P-E-C-T myself.
(Aretha said it best!)

In this way, our life flows back and forth, from the inner to the outer, from the world back to us. We are constantly reaching out to the world and bringing our experiences in to process them. When we infuse all that we process with our new understanding and love of life, and we support it with our spiritual practices, our life force, our Shakti, grows. Then we begin to make a difference, just by our presence.

When it comes to nurturing our spirit we have an abundance of personal choices, all of them doors leading to the soul. Whatever one we choose, it is important that our spiritual life enhance our own sense of well-being, and the well-being of those around us. Nurturing our spirit may begin as small acts of giving to ourselves, but eventually, by connecting with our inner life, we offer all that we have to others.

The 5 Principles of Ageless Living

It is only when we feel we are spiritually nurtured that we feel the confidence and calm to go even deeper within.

nature *is* nurture

The first step to nurturing our spirit is to realize that spirit is in us and around us all the time, whether we are aware of it or not. Spirituality can be found in very simple things: the awesomeness of nature, the unexpected kindness of a stranger, the smile or touch of your partner, the exuberant joy of a child. If you have any doubt that you have the ability to connect with God or others, think of how you received the world's wonders when you were a child. Children honor and respect the spirit of nature and its beauty because they understand it instinctively. Birds, flowers, insects, and butterflies are often the first things that evoke joyful cries of recognition in children. Try to approach the world with the openness of a child. Take pleasure in the sights, sounds, and smells that greet your senses. You will begin to find yourself rediscovering the essentials within your spirit and the spirit of the world around you.

> *To know even one life has breathed easier because you have lived. This is the meaning of success.*
> —RALPH WALDO EMERSON

When my daughter, Ryan, was young, I often had her put her arms around a tree and hug it. Sometimes we would do it together, stretching our arms around the trunk from both sides, our fingers straining to meet each other's. I encouraged her to look up and see the height of the branches above us and to imagine the length of the roots stretching out beneath us. We could both feel the vastness of nature and the closeness of the connection to each other. She says that today because of those experiences she finds that when she goes out into nature "things just get better."

Recently, it struck Ryan that she is passing on that feeling of connection to nature to her three-year-old son, Jaden. As soon as he could walk she taught him to respect nature, explaining that if he rips a leaf or a bud off a flower the plant has feelings and might be hurt. If an "offering" of a flower did end up in his tiny hand, he ceremoniously bent over to "kiss it better." Once Ryan asked him, "Why don't we swing at the plants with your sword?" he solemnly replied, "Because it hurts them." At three, he already has a sense of the importance of honoring all forms of life. Maybe this is the simplest way to understand why we need to nurture our spirit at every age: to feel the unity and empathy that remind us we are part of the whole.

Taking a beautiful walk in the woods is one of my favorite things to do, both to honor my body and to nurture my

> *Be really whole and all things will come to you.*
>
> —LAO-TZU

spirit. Walking in nature gives me the chance to see what the seasons are offering, to break from my routine, and to connect to what is natural: the soaring trees that offer shade from up above, the lush, new-green spring leaves shimmering in the sunlight, the splashes of color from vivid, scented flowers. Nature is alive, pulsating with all its sights and sounds, and all of nature knows exactly what it is supposed to be doing. It is only we who become out of sync with the natural flow. Bombarded daily by the sounds that accompany our busy lives—cars honking, ambulances whining, machines whirling, alarms buzzing, computers clicking—good heavens, our frazzled nerves need a break! When we spend time in nature, we connect back to its soothing, natural flow, allowing it to caress our sorry nerves and restore us to health. It doesn't matter if we are in a park or a garden, in the mountains or by the sea. Nature soothes our brow and sends us back home refreshed.

Experiencing tranquillity in nature, we reach to match its serenity and in doing so, we too become serene. Nature sets a standard. It speaks to us, and we echo it back. When we experience beauty in nature, we are raised to its level. I found this out during a recent visit to California when my friend Reece took me to the giant redwoods of Muir Woods in Marin County. Feeling stressed from the demands of life and the stimulus of the city, I was grateful to be surrounded by the power of Mother Nature. I felt it immediately. The silence hit me first. I was enveloped in stillness that towered 250 feet above. As I reverently walked among the giant redwoods, I felt I was in the presence of great spirits, that I was in nature's church. I saw perfection in those trees. I felt awe for their five-hundred-year-old wisdom, and gently my soul was calmed. Standing there, amid the grandeur of such spiritual beauty, I felt reassured, confident in the order of life around me. And I understood why delegates from all over the world came together after World War II to draft and sign the charter of the United Nations among these giant redwoods. Their choice of such a spiritually healing place and their decision to use the surroundings as a backdrop to form a union among nations showed me just how powerfully nurturing nature can be.

Most new discoveries are suddenly seen things that were always there.
—SUSANNE K. LANGER

live large and true

When we nurture our spirit and strengthen our connection to all of life, we want to protect it. We understand that we are all one, and we realize that any harm we may do to another living creature we really do to ourselves. A true life and a rich spiritual life encourages us to connect with those around us with a wonderful feeling of *oneness*. When we detach from the truth of that oneness, we feel disconnected, cut off from the spiritual benefits that can be ours. Whether we realize it or not, we are all connected—no matter our race or gender or any of the other categories we put ourselves and others into. We are at our best when we act from a larger spiritual perspective. Our hearts open, we become capable of great love for one another, and we become our most noble, most honorable selves. And when we feel that opening of our heart, we also feel greater love for ourselves. Our life takes on new meaning when we live large and true. We expand our vision when we nurture our spirit, and we are filled with compassion. We become kinder, more patient, more forgiving toward others and ourselves.

At midlife we are in the unique position to realize that by developing more meaning in our life we have the power to affect and change the world around us. We aren't willing to accept things at face value now—if we ever were. Every woman I speak with expresses a need for deeper understanding at this time in her life, a need for a more complete role for herself, and for more meaning in her relationships. When we were younger and thinking about making our mark in life, chances are our focus was different, more concerned with achievement than with reflection. But things change, thank God. And now, as we get older, we have a deeper need for more soulful pursuits, for a life with a larger and more generous outlook. We have a desire to *complete* ourselves (if such a thing is possible), and we want to live a life that is thoughtful, balanced, kind, and true.

Our relationships only get better with a strong inner life. My friends tell me how much their relationships with their partners improve from the insights that come when they focus on their own spiritual needs. Some of them even say that the more time they spend nurturing their spirit, the better their relationships are with everyone they are close to.

A single act of kindness throws out roots in all directions, and the roots spring up and make new trees.

—AMELIA EARHART

When we take the time to look at life through a spiritual lens we are able to see our own part in the grand scheme of things. We see that apparent coincidences aren't coincidences at all, that our problems happen for a reason. Every difficulty brings us some form of reward: wisdom, growth, understanding, transformation. And when we truly grasp this, we see the true nature of living a large spiritual life.

Any time we come into contact with someone for even the smallest shared moment—the grocery store cashier, the bus driver, the mail carrier—any time we connect with other people, we have the opportunity to make ordinary interactions, however fleeting, uplifting. Amid the stress of day-to-day living, all we really need is a series of very small inspiring moments to turn an okay day into a good day, and a good day into a great one. My friend Hilton says that a simple change in outlook is what makes the daily routine special. A day, he says, is made up of a thousand ordinary moments, and we each have the ability to make those moments extraordinary.

A spiritual life transforms our mundane moments into magic ones. It makes simple circumstances sacred. It takes chance meetings and turns them into potential revelations. With a spiritual outlook we never know who is going to come into our life holding a piece of the puzzle. We never know what truth will announce itself next. With a spiritual outlook, we have a sense of anticipation and joy. There is potential in each moment when we live in this way. The stresses of day-to-day life don't have to diminish our inner joy and make us feel contracted or small. When we exist on only one level, mechanically fulfilling problem-oriented tasks all day long, we begin to question our worth. That's when the noise of the world can drown out the voice of God.

tune in

I know it can be hard for busy women to embrace the idea of nourishing a spiritual life, especially if they haven't paid close attention to it before. I also know that some women don't feel the need. During a recent talk I saw this clearly when I asked a large group of women to write down how they would rank the importance of nurturing their spirit on a scale from one to ten, one being "not at all" and ten being "most of all." Of the women who ranked nurturing their spirit as "one"—not at all important—almost all said the reason was that they had no time. How sad.

Women especially are asked to give and give and give. But without finding ways to fill ourselves back up again we will, sooner or later, have nothing left to give. Who nurtures the nurturer? You can go to the well only so many times before it eventually runs dry. Eastern wisdom says that when you are constantly focused on the outside world, over time you will become empty. You will lose the *rasa*, or the "juice" of life. So we must find opportunities, even in little ways, to develop and take care of our inner life, to replenish our *rasa*. Think of it. If our inner life becomes an emotional afterthought, where will we go to replenish ourselves? How will we find our inner joy? How will we fill up the well? Truthfully, it doesn't take time; it takes *awareness*. And if we don't develop the awareness of how simple joys can nurture us we will never have the inner resources to take us through life's challenges.

My friend Patricia had been trying to get her mother to slow down for years, to take time for herself, to pamper and nurture herself. Her mother's answer was always, "I will, later on. I don't have time now." Her mother recently had a stroke, leaving her incapacitated and unable to speak. After years of putting off taking care of herself because she thought she had no time, as Patricia sadly says, "All my mother has now *is* time."

Ignoring our inner life and postponing our spiritual development can lead to unnecessary stress and exhaustion, or worse. Take the time to nurture your spirit, before it's too late. We are spiritual beings who need to be in touch with our core and we can neglect ourselves only so far before we ultimately crack. Sometimes it takes a trauma to know our true essence. But we don't have to wait for something so extreme.

We can find comfort in knowing that a life lesson can hide within our suffering. But to save our spiritual life for a rainy day of the soul is to shortchange ourselves on the sunny days.

When we're not in balance things happen in our life to "right" us. Life sends us small signals that we are off course. We need to be aware and heed them, or life will give us larger lessons until we do. These signs can be subtle at first: our instincts may signal that something isn't quite right. We may meet a series of uncanny "coincidences," or we may experience a series of small events that don't turn out as we intended. Whatever it is, we need to tune in to this dialogue and hear the truth. Only then can we make the proper adjustments and shift our course. In my experience, life works this way.

So how do we tune in? By making turning inward a regular practice. Going within, through activities such as meditation, yoga, or spending time in nature, gives us the opportunity to hear a deeper voice, a more truthful voice. And over time we hear the truth. In the quiet of spiritual pursuits we can create little pockets of calm during our day, cushions to buffer the pressures of day-to-day life. We can feed our spirit and renew our optimism.

Life isn't just "stuff" that happens to us. Everything we experience is there to help us evolve.

I know that when I take the time to turn inward with a yoga class, for example, I am infused with energy, yet very relaxed and calm. From this quiet place, I find it much easier to solve problems and deal with stress. When I pause during my day and stop to meditate I find that answers to questions I've struggled with come more easily because I am connected to a great reservoir of universal knowledge that I believe we all have inside. And when I spend time outdoors, enjoying nature's perfection, I return to my daily duties refreshed. I let go of the mental chatter, breathe, and find my own natural rhythm. I feel more centered, more loving, and self-aware.

Some women have told me that they question the

value of spending the little free time they have on spiritual activities. Although I know it is challenging, we do need to find the time to turn inward. I'm always trying to look for new ways to *steal* back time for myself, time that otherwise might be frittered away. When I take back that extra twenty minutes I might have spent reading the newspaper, lingering over my second cup of cappuccino, chattering on the phone, or zoning out over my favorite TV rerun, I can then make time for my spiritual activities, even if it's only ten minutes a day.

At the end of our lives, how do we want to look upon the life we have lived?

Many women in our generation neglect spirituality because we don't see its inherent relevance to our daily lives. What we may forget is that a spiritual life is not separate from our daily lives; it is in *how* we live our daily lives. When we lose sight of this, I imagine God sitting up there wondering about us. "What's this? She never calls, she never writes?" Besides supporting the belief that everything and everyone has a purpose, that there is a divine plan and we are an important part of it, a full inner life makes us beautiful. When we are fueled by our inner life our spirit shines through us, to our partner, our family and friends, and to the world. Our inner light resonates outward, as beauty. Only through nurturing our spirit can we realize our *true* beauty and live our true life.

the way in

Finding quiet moments to nurture our spirit is imperative at midlife. We need to "check in," to regularly ask ourselves how we are doing, how we are feeling. It's important to retreat and regain an inner calm, even if it's only for a short time. There are many ways to nurture your spirit, and there is no wrong way. What's important is that we make the effort to put aside a regular time when we can make an inner connection. By turning inward we reconnect to our source so that we infuse all that we do with our individual magic. Find the way that brings you your own moments of calm and make that time a precious part of your everyday living.

meditation

Meditating can change your life. It can quickly lead the body to a more relaxed physical state, lower your blood pressure, slow your heartbeat, increase oxygen circulation, reduce muscle tension, improve your immune system, and calm your mind. When I meditate daily, my life is different. The events of my day run more smoothly. I have the insights I need to solve problems and I have a much calmer and clearer viewpoint during even my most stressful moments. Meditation and the understanding that spirituality brings have changed how I view just about everything. I have meditated for many years now, and over time, I've been able to see the positive influence this practice has had on my life.

Hundreds of years ago, Patanjali, a great sage and the father of Yoga, wrote that "meditating was the stilling of the thought waves of the mind." From this place of restored serenity, we come back to our daily duties refreshed. We have an expanded view of the meaning of life and our purpose in it. The more we meditate, the greater our understanding becomes and the more we fill up the inner well. Then the magic starts. We begin to create something sublime from the everyday. Our life just starts to look and feel better.

> *The only journey is the one within.*
> —RAINER MARIA RILKE

Meditating is very simple. You need only to wear loose-fitting clothes, remove your shoes, and find a quiet spot in your home where there is not too much traffic. Try to meditate in the same place each time, because that will build up a calm meditative energy, making it easier each time to go within. You may want to light incense or a candle to make your space more special. Incense creates a sensory memory that helps draw us inside. I particularly like the scent of sandalwood found in Blue Pearl or Nag Champa incense. It's less soapy and sweet than most incense.

You may also want to place objects or photos that have a spiritual meaning to you in your meditating space.

Traditionally, you would sit on a small woolen mat that is only used for meditating. This helps hold the energy. Everything in your meditation area should be honored, as it makes your experience even more sacred.

Some scents encourage calm, while others promote vitality and energy. Sandalwood and frankincense soothe us and pull us inward. Tibetan monks use them for meditating, and also in religious ceremonies. Scents like rosewood, geranium, lavender, and neroli help calm our fears and ease our anxieties.

Citrus scents can provide stimulation after meditating. Try orange, lemon, or lime. And for a quick lift, place a few drops of orange blossom oil on a cotton ball and inhale. Peppermint and spearmint can be stimulating too.

once you have set up your space, you can begin

1   Sit upright on your meditation mat with your legs folded. (If this is physically challenging, you may sit in a chair, with both feet flat on the ground.)

2   Lengthen your spine and close your eyes.

3   With your thumb and forefinger touching each other, place your hands on your knees or in your lap, one on top of the other.

THE 5 PRINCIPLES OF AGELESS LIVING

4   Take three full breaths through your nose, filling up
    your lower diaphragm and slowly letting it out, again
    through the nose.

5   Imagine your spine lengthening from the base to the
    top of your head, with each breath.

6   Now breathe regularly, always through the nose,
    watching your breath go in and go out.

7   Watch your breath enter your body. See where it goes
    inside, then watch it go out of the body.

8   Notice the space between each breath and focus on it.

9   If you are distracted by a thought, gently bring your
    mind back to your breathing and start once more to
    watch the in-breath, then the out-breath.

Remember, you want to be gentle with your mind. It will want
to do what it does best, and that is to think. You may find yourself worrying about a bill you forgot to pay or a conversation
you should have had, or even going over your laundry list.
Don't be discouraged. This is normal. When you become aware
that you are thinking and not meditating, without opening
your eyes gently bring your attention back to the breath, going
in and out. You will get back into it. Eventually, as your body
understands what you are doing, meditating will become eas-

ier to enter into. Remember to be gentle and patient with yourself; there is no such thing as a bad meditation.

Even if you can only manage to sit for meditation for a few minutes at a time, you will be doing some good to yourself and your body. As you get used to meditating regularly, you can gradually increase the length of your session. You may want to use a timer—that takes the guesswork out of it—and increase your meditation to twenty and forty-five minutes. And you want to put in some meditation time every day. That way it becomes a part of your life and you can very quickly see its positive results.

The duty of the mind is to think and we don't want to stop it. We want to go beyond it.

The quiet early morning hours are the most auspicious for meditating—between 4 A.M. and 6:30 A.M.—but some people prefer the evening before they go to bed. Only you can determine your best time for meditating. Just remember that meditating can be very relaxing, so if you do meditate at bedtime, make sure you don't confuse the two activities and fall asleep.

It's difficult to explain the wonderful, positive effects meditation can have if you haven't yet experienced it. But I can confidently say that meditating regularly over time will improve your life. As little as five or ten minutes can have a powerful effect on how smoothly your day flows, and meditating for longer periods will transform you forever.

THE 5 PRINCIPLES OF AGELESS LIVING

If you're not ready to meditate, set aside some time each day just to think, to contemplate the day or maybe your place in the world. Contemplation can be one of the mainstays of a rich, full life. It can reveal our mistakes to us, as well as show us where we've been successful. When we take the time to thoughtfully examine what happens in our life, we learn so much about ourselves. We can become aware of our patterns and tendencies. We can figure out why certain people are in our lives and discover what we need to learn from them. Best of all, we can detach our thoughts and emotions from our actions, and understand—*really* understand—what guides us. Make room in your life for some quiet contemplation and you'll be surprised at the breathtaking insights you can unearth. Just ten peaceful minutes a day can provide you with a wonderful spiritual perspective on what's really going on in your life.

The ceaseless chattering of the mind is comparable to the disturbed waters of a lake after a storm. The lake is still agitated, the water still churning so that you can't see the bottom. The debris from the tempest has muddied the water, making it brown and dirty. But once the storm has died down, the contents of the lake slowly settle to the bottom and once more the water becomes even and clear. Calm is restored. This is what meditation does to the mind. It helps us to go past the ceaseless chatter and beyond, to the calm that is deep inside each of us and can only be reached by going within.

One of the marvelous things about midlife is that it gives us a larger outlook. We realize now what's worthwhile. We can see the difference between what is fleeting and what endures, and we can appreciate the greater consequences of our actions. So often when we think of a spiritual life we think of it in opposition to a life of action, but in fact that's not true at all. Everything we do speaks of our beliefs. Our conduct is generated by our spiritual viewpoint because what we hold to be true ultimately manifests itself in our actions. Contemplation reminds us that things don't happen in a vacuum, that there are larger consequences to our actions, and that those actions are governed by our beliefs.

Your conduct is your life's legacy.

One of the most beautiful things about midlife is that it delivers us to a vantage point of wisdom where we can realize that most things aren't good or bad in themselves so much as they bring the *opportunity* to do good or bad. Taking the time to contemplate, we can embrace this truth and let go of the fear that holds us back. Think of it: there is nothing to hold us back from realizing our own greatness, and the greatness of others. Every act, every person, every relationship, every event in our life has the potential to be positive—it's up to us to recognize that potential and to do what we can to bring it to light. That's not to say that the opportunities we may be presented with will be the ones we thought we wanted. And that's not to say that it's going to be easy.

THE 5 PRINCIPLES OF AGELESS LIVING

We often have to work at bringing goodness into our lives, and to recognize goodness even when it's shrouded in difficulty. But we can do it. And both meditation and contemplation can help.

finding spirit through giving

One of the most important things in life is to feel that we can make a difference, to feel that our life is valuable and that we are needed. Women at midlife have so much to give. What better way than to give of ourselves? We can shop for seniors who have trouble getting around. We can sort donated clothes at a women's shelter. We can read to sick children. We can sit with hospice patients. There are so many ways to give, so many opportunities. From the single random act of kindness to the ongoing volunteer commitment, we can realize how much we all need each other. And on a more subtle level, we may wonder who is really being given to? It may not be so obvious.

Giving makes us feel good. That is not the reason to do it, of course, but the lift we get when we give of ourselves is immeasurable. We nurture our spirit both by giving and with the good feeling that giving brings. We do not necessarily need to give money. What may be more valuable is to give of our time, our organizational skills, our creativity, or simply our compassion.

During one Christmas season, I passed the church on my street and saw the homeless men and women staking out an early spot for the evening. As I noticed a man sleeping on the bare sidewalk without even a cover over him to keep out the cold, I was struck anew by the enormity of what I had in my own life. I made up my mind then and there to help.

I went home and ordered a number of below-zero sleeping bags. When they arrived, along with a friend, I prepared piping hot soup and some food, and we set about giving them out. The word got out quickly that hot food was on its way and the reception was heartwarming. I had the wonderful opportunity that night to meet people I will never forget. Clutching a cheap furniture cover, one man named Ola turned down the brand-new sleeping bag I offered. "Please give it to someone who is more needy. I have this," he said proudly, showing me his old boiled-wool blanket. Speaking in Italian with another man, I discovered to my surprise and delight that he grew up in the same small town in Italy that I had visited. Later in the evening I was approached by a well-dressed woman who had been watching us. I assumed she too was a volunteer until she tentatively asked me if I could please find her some milk to drink. These small exchanges gave me a glimpse into lives that

Small acts become great gifts when someone needs us.

THE 5 PRINCIPLES OF AGELESS LIVING

I would otherwise never have known. They were a gift for me, and I will never be able to walk past that church indifferently again. We tend to believe that it is the big acts in life that have the greatest impact, but I believe that even *small* acts of kindness make a difference. The gift of self is the most precious gift we have to give. Life is at its most beautiful when our ability to give meets someone's truest need.

tai chi

The ancient Chinese practice of tai chi (pronounced "ty chee") is a gentle exercise that can both strengthen and nurture our spirit. It is made up of thirteen postures that get our "good" energy flowing, increasing our strength and resistance to "negative" energy.

When we are healthy, our life force, or chi, flows through us freely and we feel fully alive. When we are stressed, our energy becomes blocked; we feel tired, depressed, out of balance, or even just a little bit "off." Because our body is a system of integrated parts, when chi is blocked in one area, we feel the imbalance all over. The slow movements of tai chi calm us, bringing harmony to our body, and a feeling of being in sync with the world.

My friend Sharon is a personal trainer and an Olympic medalist in fencing, a very high-stress sport. Her

BENEFITS OF TAI CHI

- *Relaxes the mind and body, reducing stress*

- *Increases flexibility*

- *Prevents fatigue and helps concentration*

- *Improves balance and coordination*

- *Strengthens the immune system*

husband, Mike, an Olympic decathlete and also a trainer, was concerned about all the pressure she was under, and wanted to find a more peaceful way for her to exercise, something that would help create some calm in her life. They found it in tai chi. At first Sharon muscled her way through all the movements the same way she attacked her fencing. But she kept at it, and with practice was able to let down her guard. It took her a couple of weeks, but finally Sharon found herself starting to relax, flowing into the poses. In time, she allowed herself to be calmed by the slow, meditative movements, ultimately giving herself over to the poise and strength of this ancient practice. Now in her forties and the mother of twins, Sharon uses tai chi as a gentle and efficient exercise to keep herself in harmony and in shape, and to connect to her inner life.

music

A beautiful piece of music can soothe our frazzled nerves. When I come home after a long day, I immediately put on a calming piece of music. Music nurtures us by changing our mood, soothing our agitation, and making us more receptive to beauty, harmony, peacefulness, and generosity. Music takes us to another world. Even when our senses are on overload, harmonious music finds its way into our heart. It transforms us, taking us to a sweeter level, helping us feel that everything is right in the world.

Every great artist creates out of a higher state. When we are receptive to their art, we too are transported to that state. We soar. Music lets us access spirit through sound. A great piece of work encourages us to expand as we listen, and we too become great. Music vibrates through our whole being and brings into harmony all our jangled pieces. Music is healing. It brings us into connection with our inner self. It makes us feel.

Music has had an extraordinary impact on my life. I was very lucky that my mother loved the classics and played them in our home daily. When I was very little, not yet five, I experienced music as something visual. I *saw* music; I *saw* the notes dance in the air and I couldn't sit still. I had to follow the shape of the notes with my hands and body. My parents thought I had dance abilities, but I was just expressing my soul. Great music has always connected me with spirit.

Music gives us immediate access to our soul. When we hear Beethoven's "Ninth" we feel grand, larger than life. Mozart's gaiety and lightness ripple over us like a brook. The haunting melody of Albinoni's "Adaggio" reaches directly to our heart, moving us to compassion. And the stunning rhythms of Gloria Gaynor's "I Will Survive" convince us we can do anything! I like to find pieces that enhance my mood: the lightness of Vivaldi to complement dinner; upbeat fifties pop songs like "Splish, Splash," when I'm taking a bath (really!); and the joyous seventies music of ABBA, if I want a general lift. On Sunday afternoons, anything by Mozart will rejuvenate my spirit. Or, if I'm in a meditative state, I'll put on a CD of sitar music that will draw me inside for meditation. I often play soothing chants in the background throughout the day. Many people say they feel incredibly relaxed, almost meditative, when they step into my apartment. I attribute that to the healing music I continually play.

Eastern sages believe that certain music resonates with us because it re-creates the sounds of nature and spirit, sounds

You are the music while the music lasts.

—T. S. ELIOT

that draw us to the deepest parts of our being. Listening intently to sounds in nature—the sea, the wind, the popping of fire—can clear our mind of worldly concerns. Music that re-creates these natural sounds is said to have the same effect. The meditation teacher Swami Chidvilasananda writes, "The deep call of the conch mimics the ocean; the rumble of drums, the earth; the tinkle of bells echoes the wind; and the clash of cymbals represents the crackle of fire." When we bring this music into our daily life, and focus our mind on really listening, then music adds a spiritual dimension, opening us to the nurturing it brings.

gardening

Working with the earth and making things grow brings us a sense of satisfaction and a feeling of oneness. When we are continually surrounded by man-made things—computers, telephones, faxes, cars, and household appliances—we can feel cut off from spiritual nourishment. Returning to the land, actually feeling the earth between our fingers, can connect us to the natural order of things and bring us into harmony with our self.

As far back as I can remember I have gardened. When I was a child, my parents infused in me a love of all growing things. Recently, when traveling so much for work had left me depleted, I had the urge to nourish myself by feeling the earth again. With my friend Elizabeth, who shares my passion for gardening, I plunged into a garden project. We tied tomatoes to their training sticks and foraged through her herb garden to select seasonings for our meals. We planted new rosebushes along the pathways and, as a special project, we selected a red one for our friend Regina, a pink one for our friend Michele, and a white one for me. Elizabeth wanted to plant these lovely roses in the name of each of her friends so that she could think of us as she watched each rosebush grow. This loving and generous task brought joy to my heart. I finally began to relax, to feel more in balance. The world started to slow down, and I found myself listening to another, deeper rhythm, feeling one with nature and myself.

It is only when you start a garden that you realize something important happens every day.

—Geoffrey B. Charlesworth

I love to get up in the morning and see what has developed in the garden overnight. I never cease to be amazed by nature's generosity. I especially adore roses. The deep red buds promise lush blooms, and I *ooh* and *ahh* over each vivid offering. I feel that roses transform themselves every day and I revel in their sudden transitions. Their perfection moves me to "request" permission before I cut each bloom, gently laying my treasures in my worn straw basket.

Through nature I see before me the miracle of life appear and reappear, over and over again, and I am continually renewed. I experience a connection in the garden, and that connection is spiritual.

sacred spaces

To me, outward chaos and inward confusion go hand in hand. When my living space and workspace are overly busy and disorganized, *I* feel overly busy and disorganized. That's why I like to devise a sacred space, a place to keep my mind clear, a place that leaves me better prepared to tap into my wisdom and contemplate. When we understand that contemplate means "to create space for the divine to enter," we can also recognize how important that space can be to our well-being.

Creating a private, sacred space is one of the most loving acts you can do for yourself. Whether it is indoors or out, and whether you find yourself drawn to meditation, yoga, journaling, or other rituals, give yourself a place that will set the scene for your spiritual contemplation and practices. You can place pictures or postcards of nature scenes in your sacred space, arrange cut flowers or plants—anything that inspires you to nourish your inner life. You may also want to play a chant or nature's music; sounds of the ocean, a rain forest, or birdsongs. I love to hear the calming sounds of a sitar or tamboura calling me inside, but of course it's what you want (and need!) that's important here. Just make your space special—and your own—and you will be continually drawn "home" to rejuvenate.

I know some women who have created wonderful personal spaces out of practically nothing. My friend Barbara transformed a tiny spare closet into her quiet space. She set up a small altar with some objects that were meaningful to her, such as a tiny photograph of herself at age five to remind her where she had come from. She retreats to her space to contemplate, to meditate, and to become calm. Another friend, Kandy, who is a talented architect, built her sacred space especially for meditation. Her space is honored—shoes are left outside the door—and she has a beautiful chant softly playing twenty-four hours a day. Whenever I enter into her candlelit meditating room I am enveloped in a powerful blanket of calm and am immediately pulled into a deep, peaceful tranquillity.

My friend's sister needed a special room to heal her after her divorce. She set out to create the most beautiful room she had ever seen, one she remembered from a childhood trip to New York's Frick Museum. On the museum's

Learn to get in touch with the silence within yourself and know that everything in this life has a purpose.

—ELISABETH KÜBLER-ROSS

THE 5 PRINCIPLES OF AGELESS LIVING

Web site, she found a "virtual walk-through tour." A few clicks later, she found *the room!* Remembering how she loved the goddess Venus, she clicked on another site and discovered a wall-size mural of Botticelli's *Birth of Venus.* Voilà. Her Goddess Room was born. In her special space, she says, every awakening is a "rebirth," every night an act of gratitude.

In my sacred space, I have small objects that I brought back from India: a bell with a beautiful sound that I like to ring, an incense holder, some semiprecious stones, and small photographs of great sages. Each of my objects is on a beautiful piece of Indian silk. It's a place I honor and love; it's where I meditate. My sacred space is a small, cherished area. It's an area that inspires me and feeds my spirit. Whether your own space is ornate or simple, we all need a place to take a breath. Your sacred space then becomes your spirit made manifest.

Make Room

Let your imagination guide you to create your personal haven from the world, or even just from your household. Make it a gentle place with well-chosen but minimal *stuff*—clutter can make us feel chaotic. Natural objects, like a stone, minerals, or a special shell, are especially soothing because they bring us closer to the earth. Lighting a candle can also help create a ritual to make our sacred space unique.

as the spirit moves you

We think of movement as being good for the body, but movement can also be good for the soul, helping you to connect to and nurture your spirit. When I get my body moving, my spirit is lifted. I feel especially renewed when I'm active while enjoying nature. My favorite activity of all is walking. It gives me the exercise I need, and at the same time, allows me to commune with nature. As my friends the respected yoga pioneers Ila and Garrett Sarley say in their wonderful book *Walking Yoga*, walking can be a "flow of meditative movement."

My "gym" is Central Park—that's where I exercise with my workout partner, Mike. He takes me to unique areas within the park for my regular workouts. One morning, while I diligently did the "dead bug" exercise for my tummy muscles, I spied the perfect birds' nest tucked under the leaves high above me. As I strained to complete my set, I delighted in following the developments of the bird family as they tended their nest. Then, as I held one of my stretches, Mike pointed out a woman returning a wayward turtle to the pond. A little later, while performing my step-ups on one of the park benches, I watched a pair of male and female ducks glide from one side of the lake to another, leaving a silver stream in their wake. I took in all the beauty around me. Then, wanting to prolong the moment, I asked myself, "What else am I perceiving?" And I realized that just below my consciousness I had been hearing birds singing; feeling cool, sensual breezes along my bare arms; noticing lush, wet leaves waving to me. All this richness was available to me while I exercised. I just had to open myself to it.

You don't have to move fast or exercise hard to receive nature's benefits. I spent time learning to fly-fish at my friend Cathy's ranch in Colorado, and I became focused on catching my fish to the exclusion of all else. Concentrating on a specific spot I was aiming for, I felt only the perfection of the moment. Hours passed in a meditative state. All sense of time was lost. I knew only that I had been communing with nature and that nature had somehow been communing with me. Fishing became a form of meditation for me. Yes, I was engaged in physical activity, but I was also feeding my soul.

Riding a bike, cross-country skiing, and skating are just some of the other activities that allow us to breathe fresh air and be part of nature's perfection. There is something about using our bodies in the outdoors that especially nurtures our spirit. Golfing, too, places us in a calm setting, no matter how intense the competition.

My friend Claude Lelouch maintains that you don't have to go all the way to India to have the benefits of meditation. You can gain a definitive philosophy of life, he says, just by riding a bike. On the flat roads, he explains, you're relaxed and free, taking in everything around you, just as in life when everything is going great. Ahead, you see a steep incline. Like all challenges, you don't want to attack it right away; you prepare for the right time. Then, by the time you reach the mountain you are ready to strike. Riding a bike is like life, Claude says; you have to know your timing. I found that biking revealed my habit of preparing too early for "the obstacle" ahead. By the time we got to the mountain, we were laughing: I had already exhausted myself!

One of my friends took up golfing in her fifties because, she said, it combined walking, visiting with her friends, and a perfect lawn that someone else had to mow.

I think of exercise outdoors as a *twofer*. You can get two payoffs for the price of one— as at Wal-Mart. Exercise benefits our body *and* connects us with nature, nurturing our spirit.

spirit in art

Museums and galleries are wonderful places to nurture our spirit. When we contemplate great art, we see something created from a higher state, and we are drawn, naturally, to the same level. When we see a Michelangelo or a Botticelli, it connects with us inside in a way that moves us beyond simple appreciation of the work itself.

I will never forget my mother's reaction upon seeing Michelangelo's *David* for the first time. As we approached the room the statue was in, I whispered, "Mom, prepare yourself." I heard her gasp as the *David* came into view. She didn't speak, but I noticed a tear trickle down her cheek. Later, she confided to me that in that moment she *couldn't* speak; she was so overwhelmed by the statue's perfection, nothing could prepare her for its impact. It was a spiritual moment for both of us.

For me, Michelangelo's *The Prisoners* evokes a kind of churchlike awe. The half-formed, giant beings, pushing their way out of the marble, seem to breathe the stone alive with their presence. Michelangelo has said that the men already existed inside the stone, he just had to remove the excess. It is magical to me that an artist can give us this experience hundreds of years later, and that his genius can make us feel the form in the formless.

I have stood transfixed before da Vinci's *Annunciation*, overwhelmed by Fra Angelico's religious murals, intrigued by the knowingness and simplicity of Mona Lisa's smile. And I was uplifted. An inner shift took place in that moment; even though communicated from the artist years and years ago, communication on a spiritual level is timeless.

Monet's *Water Lilies*, Van Gogh's *Starry Night*, the Sistine Chapel, the Coliseum, the *Pietà*, the Elgin Marbles, the Parthenon—great works offer us an opportunity to transform ourselves. We feel awe, we feel wonder, we feel mystery. Before such greatness, we know there must be a God in the universe. Great art, created by spirit, and moving *our* spirit. Here we are today, spirit connecting with spirit.

Beauty in all forms, whether in art, furniture, or literature, nurtures our spirit. There is art to be found almost everywhere; we have only to seek it out. We can find it in the simplicity of a one-room country church and in the massive structures of big-city buildings. We can admire it in well-made desk objects and in the grandeur of a national land-mark. We can discover it in an enchanted backyard garden and in the harmony of a friend's living room. We can be mesmerized by Shakespeare's sonnets, and still charmed by *The Velveteen Rabbit.*

Anyone who keeps the ability to see beauty never grows old.

—FRANZ KAFKA

Beauty in the simplest of forms speaks to us. Whenever we can, wherever we look, if we take the time to marvel at human creativity, we feed our souls.

rituals

Rituals can add such value to our everyday acts. As tools to enhance our *sadhana*—our spiritual work on ourselves—rituals can add significance, honor, and fun to whatever we do. Rituals make everything we do more special. Often we think of them as being reserved for holidays or religious occasions, but to me, rituals transform an ordinary event into something unique.

THE 5 PRINCIPLES OF AGELESS LIVING

Rituals imbue our actions with greater meaning, making them more important, more significant, more magical. Any act can become sacred with a ritual. When we say a prayer, when we light a candle, when we give thanks, we take an extra step to honor what we are about to undertake. Rituals are especially helpful for someone who is beginning to find his or her spiritual focus. Burning incense while we meditate, playing chants that draw us inside, or surrounding ourselves with photos or objects that remind us of a higher state—all can signal that it is time to go within.

The soul is here for its own joy.

—RUMI

Patanjali, the great author of yoga aphorisms, writes in *How to Know God*, one of my favorite books, that rituals are an "excellent training for the wandering mind of the beginner. Each successive act recalls the mind to the thought behind the act. You're too busy to think of anything else. Thought and action, action and thought, form a continuous chain and it is amazing to find what a comparatively high degree of concentration you can achieve even from the very first. Also, ritual gives you a sense of serving God in a very direct but intimate manner."

Patanjali goes on to say that, in spirituality, sometimes we try to grasp concepts that are beyond the mind, and when we use simple things—like flowers, incense, or other rituals and offerings—it makes it easier to focus.

At midlife, as we look to fulfill our need for ways to better honor life and living, rituals can be very helpful. We are wiser now. We know that we need to feel connected and we want to infuse our activities from a deeper place. Rituals help us make that connection. My friend Michele, who does wonderful healing work, helps others develop their inner lives. She is often called upon to create a ritual to bless a new home. This ceremony honors, purifies, and blesses the new living space, *and* creates excitement for the new homeowners. It heightens their anticipation, creating a magic about starting life in their new home.

Mealtime Blessing

Bless this food I am about to eat. I thank the earth that offered it. I thank all those that made it possible for it to be before me. I offer this food to the highest.

But we don't have to wait for a special occasion to benefit from a ritual. We can create one at every opportunity. Say blessings before a meal, play special music while vacuuming the house, wave incense or sage to "clean" a room, ask for blessings before tackling a work assignment. There are so many ways we can honor a place, a project, or a simple routine. Remember Mary Tyler Moore as Mary Richards? She brought a red rose to work every Monday morning!

some enchanted evening

I love the ritual of an "enchanted bath." It gives me an opportunity to rest my spirit and to rejuvenate my body. Just ten minutes in my magic bath rejuvenates my soul and I feel ready to start again. Creating your own enchanted bath is filled with all the fun that bath rituals can have:

1   As you prepare to pour your bath, choose an aromatic oil to uplift and energize or one to calm and relax you. I have a friend who swears by the restorative powers of Aura Cacia Tranquility bath salts. Seek out your favorite mixture, or make your own.

Relaxing Bath Blend	*Stimulating Bath Blend*
Roman Chamomile	Rosemary Oil
Lavender Oil	Lemon Oil
Sweet Almond Oil	Lavender Oil
	Sweet Almond Oil

Add twenty-five drops to full bath or dab on wrists and temples. Experiment to find the right proportions for you.

2   Put on music that will be deeply relaxing while you
    soak. I love the soothing songs of Norah Jones and
    Diana Krall. Dim the lights and strategically place a
    few scented candles around the tub.

3   Add bubbles for fun, mineral salts for muscle relaxing,
    and a terry pillow to cushion your head.

4   Prepare a calming herb tea to sip at tubside and you
    are all ready to slide into your delicious bath.

5   After your transforming soak, wrap yourself in a cozy,
    soft robe and curl up with a good book or movie and
    a cup of tea or hot cocoa. Yum!

The ritual of an enchanted bath can help you unwind after a hectic day, or it can rev you up if you have to go back out. Either way, soaking in your magic bath will change the way you feel in just ten minutes.

yoga

Practicing yoga on a regular basis nourishes our spirit and refines our understanding of the truth. In fact, practicing yoga can actually make us wiser. Yoga shifts the way we view our life and the life around us, putting us into harmony with the world, giving us access to our wisdom, and helping us to nurture our spirit.

I have studied yoga since I was a teenager and find that not only does it give me a wonderful physical workout, it also provides me with a completely different perspective. No matter how frazzled I may be going in to class, I am a changed person when the yoga session ends. I feel that every cell in my body is sparkling and active and excited to be alive. I definitely have a shift in outlook, a much more "anything is possible" attitude. And, I have the extra bonus of feeling refreshed, centered, and calm.

Many activities can get our bodies in shape, but yoga gives much more than just a workout. One of my yoga teachers told me, "Think of a wet sponge: when you squeeze it, you ring out all the excess. Holding yoga postures actually wrings toxins out of the body." After that, the yogic breathing infuses the body with *prana*, or energy.

To be on the spiritual path we have to be physically strong. Yoga strengthens us mentally and physically so that we can continually focus on what is meaningful. Many traditions liken being on the spiritual path to being a warrior. The practice of yoga makes us like warriors, *peaceful* warriors—but powerful ones nevertheless.

Practicing yoga regularly makes us strong and prepares us for spiritual experience. And in yoga, as in all spiritual experiences, conscious breathing is vital. In meditation, we follow the breath in and out to guide us to a deeper place inside, and in yoga we use breath combined with posture to quiet and strengthen both the body and mind.

How we breathe determines the level of calm we feel. When we are under stress we breath more shallowly, and that adds to our agitation; however, simply by taking in several long, slow breaths, we can calm our mind and our body—instantly. The first thing I say to my friends when they are upset is *"Breathe!"* Immediately, their focus and calm returns. Then, and only then, can they properly address their problem.

Like water running down the path of least resistance, with yoga we flow naturally toward the path of spirituality.

We need to breathe deeply to bring oxygen to all our cells, rid the body of toxins, and energize us, but we also use breathing to help us turn inward in meditation. Peace of mind is important at midlife, and staying calm during the day becomes even more important as we get older. One of the gifts of midlife is the understanding that our attitude affects our experiences. We know now that we can't have a deep inner life without being calm and connected. Taking long, slow, deep breaths keeps us serene and centered, receptive to nurturing our spiritual life. We certainly can't have kind, loving thoughts or actions if we are angry and stressed. That is why both yoga and meditation emphasize breathing or *pranayama,* to help connect us to spirit. To remind yourself to *breathe,* do something as simple as jot yourself a note to BREATHE! wherever you'll see it.

thank you

Most of us are overburdened and underthanked. Finding creative ways to thank people uplifts both you and those to whom you show appreciation. We can never thank people enough for *all* they do. And thanking others tells them that they are seen and appreciated, even if they didn't ask for the recognition. It is the way we can let people know we are grateful for the extra effort they made, that we notice.

My dear friend Reece is so generous with his thanks that he inspires me. He thanks people for spending time with him. He thanks them for being in his life. He thanks them for any small act they do. It just makes them want to do more! "Thanks" to his example, I am more aware of the thousand and one things people do for me during a day. Now I find that thanking others can feel so good that I look for opportunities to be grateful. I've noticed that often when thanking somebody, bad behavior will switch to good as the person realizes they are being validated. Thanking is a kind of magic.

We give thanks because we are grateful for something someone has done or offered. It doesn't matter if we thank in person, or with a small gift, or one of my favorite ways, with a handwritten note. I love to collect unique cards and delicate paper and write my thank-you notes with my special fountain pen. A simple thank-you can turn a small, thoughtful gesture into a spiritual connection.

Thank you, Merci, Gracias, Ngiyabonga Dhanyabad,

To the photographer in New York who was determined to get me my first job when I was a teenager and no one wanted to hire me . . . To my friend Kandy, who kindly took me in when I had lost everything, who fed me, buoyed my spirits, and made me laugh . . . To the American Airlines agent at LaGuardia Airport who left her post, grabbed my bag, and ran with me all the way to the gate so that I wouldn't miss my plane . . . And to all of you for sharing this journey with me.

As women at midlife we've lived long enough to know the wisdom of being grateful. And we have *so much* to be grateful for. Yes, we all struggle at times. We all have sorrows and challenges, and sometimes we face despair; but that's all part of this large, wondrous gift called life. Think of the endless possibilities for joy and love in each day. Honor those possibilities and be grateful for them. Be grateful for the lessons you have learned and for what you have experienced. Be grateful for the treasures you have found in your challenges. Be grateful for your vitality and strength, and for your own tremendous spirit. Be grateful for your friends and loved ones. Be grateful for life in all its forms, and for the opportunity to participate in the world around you. Above all else, be grateful for this moment. Right here. Right now.

Principle Three:
Honor Your Body

Create Energy and Strength
for Your Best Health

Our body is our servant and companion—for life. But we so often take it for granted. We have demands and desires, and we make our trusty body follow them. We push ourselves when we are tired, we eat when we're not hungry (or we don't eat when we *are* hungry), we do too much of one thing, and not enough of another. And, as if that weren't all, most of us have a dialogue with our body that borders on the abusive. "You are so slow." "You have a fat tummy." "Boy, you're looking old." We wouldn't treat *anyone*—another person, a child, a pet—with such disregard. Why do we feel it's okay to be that way with our own dear body?

The fact is it's not okay. It's not okay to be negligent, to ignore or abuse our body, to deny support to that which supports us so faithfully. If we've gone through life without listening to what our body has been telling us, if we've forced our body forward as if driving a car at top speed without enough gas or oil, then at midlife we're going to start feeling the effects of all that "reckless driving." And, for want of a better explanation, we may be tempted to label the damage "old age" or "natural." Let's not deceive ourselves. What we may be calling old age may simply be our own carelessness and neglect. That's the bad news.

The good news? There is no reason that most of us can't have a strong, healthy body at midlife and beyond. It's not too late to turn things around. I won't say it doesn't matter what you have done to your body up to this point. Of course it matters. But what you need to know now is this: it's never too late to do the things that will help you get the body you want. If you've struggled with your weight all your life, if you've been resistant to exercise or had a difficult relationship with food, now is the time to employ that marvelous midlife perspective to finally deal with those issues. Now is the time to use your wisdom to dismantle the patterns that have held you back. Now is the time to use your confidence to accept that your body can feel strong and look good. Now is the time to honor your body and become the woman you know you can be, inside and out. *Now is the time.*

It's important to understand that the quality of life ahead of us depends on how we take care of our body *today.* When we begin to really honor our body and treat it with respect, when we take care of our body and cherish it as if it is a small, beloved child, we *will* notice a difference—very often sooner than we think. My friend Mike, an Olympic decathlete who now trains people from all walks of life, taught me a lot about the human body. He says that we can completely renew ourselves in just about three months. That's pretty good considering we may have forty years of bad habits to undo. Now that doesn't mean you can shed all those excess pounds you may have been carrying around for the past ten years, and it doesn't mean that you can eliminate all your wrinkles or grow two inches taller.

If you think of your body as a small child that needs your wise and gentle guidance, then of course you will want to tuck it under your protective wing and care for it.

What it does mean is that your muscles can be stronger, your joints can improve, your balance can be better, and your respiratory system and lung capacity can become more efficient. Your heart can be stronger, pumping more blood and creating less strain on the body. You can burn more calories, becoming slimmer and fitter. You can have more energy and more vitality. You can probably sleep better too. When your body improves, you are going to feel better all around. And that includes having a more positive approach to life!

At midlife, we go through more dramatic physical transitions than at any other time in our lives since adolescence. Even before menopause we undergo changes in our skin and hair, changes in our metabolism, changes in our bone density, changes in our moods and in our sense of well-being. We put on weight that we can't seem to lose. We get out of bed in the morning, feeling stiffer than we remember. We become winded on that extra set of stairs. We find that our eyesight isn't as sharp as it used to be, and eventually, we find ourselves giving in and buying that first pair of reading glasses. Fortunately, along with all these physical changes, midlife often brings more time to take better care of our overall health. Our children are older now and more independent (we may even be empty nesters), and it's likely that we are at a more senior point in our career, so most of us *do* have more time and attention to spend on ourselves. So what's holding us back from caring for our bodies properly?

> *We do not stop playing because we grow old. We grow old because we stop playing.*
> —ANONYMOUS

Everything we do, even unconsciously, accumulates and ends up, over time, affecting how we look and feel. Once we decide to take care of ourselves properly—a very important part of living agelessly—then we can have the energy and glowing health that supports what we want to do. When we honor our body we treat it with the tenderness that comes from understanding that it is under our care. And while that may mean realizing our own limitations, it doesn't have to mean being limited *by* them.

At this stage of my life I especially want my body to be as healthy and strong as it can be. I want to be able to do everything I want to do without my body holding me back. I want to be able to take my yoga classes, and to go biking, skiing, hiking, and swimming with my friends. I want to be strong enough to carry my own packages and bags, and run for the bus if I have to. I want to climb up several flights of stairs and not be *too* winded, and I want the flexibility to be able to switch from one to the other of my many activities without feeling the usual aches and pains. I want the vigor to keep up with my inquisitive three-year-old grandson, Jaden, and my increasingly mobile one-year-old granddaughter, Eliana, and to be attentive to my family's needs. I want to continue going on adventures with my dear friends (even if it's only to the coffee shop to catch up), and to encourage women to live their fullest lives. I want the energy and the strength to keep myself going. I want the vitality to *really* live my life.

The groundwork of all happiness is health.

—LEIGH HUNT

When I ask myself, "What do I need to accomplish these goals?" it always comes back to the same three things: eating well, exercising regularly, and making sure I get enough rest. When these three elements are part of my daily routine, all else falls into place. I know that the choices I make in each of these three areas affect me, almost immediately, in every aspect of my life. I recognize that those effects will be positive or negative depending on the choices I make. And I realize the connection between *each* choice and the way my body looks and feels.

It doesn't have to be difficult. We don't have to go to a fancy spa or spend a lot of money to honor our body. We can do it simply, one day at a time, by making better choices and gradual changes, by being mindful of our bodies' needs. We all can make good food choices, and remind ourselves that exercise is free; it's as simple as strapping on a pair of good walking shoes. If you live in the country, you have nature at your doorstep, but even in a city, you can head to a park. (But remember, window-shopping doesn't count!)

The secret of getting ahead is getting started.
—SALLY BERGER

Now is the time to use your wisdom and make the connection. Until you start to recognize how a healthful diet can keep you active, how staying active can increase your self-esteem, and how your self-esteem can affect the relationships in your life, you can't realize your full potential at every age.

All five Ageless Living Principles ask us to look at our life as a whole: our appearance, our spirit, our wisdom, our body, and our relationships. The principle Honor Your Body,

THREE STEPS TO HONORING OUR BODY

1 Eat well

2 Exercise regularly

3 Get enough rest

however, is unique in that *every-thing* in our life—how we look, how much energy we have, how healthy we feel, our sense of worth, the quality of our relationships, the love we feel in our life—is directly tied to our physical condition and our feelings about our body.

We don't need a private trainer or an expert nutrition-ist to feel our best or our healthiest. We don't have to adhere to a checklist of forbidden foods or a military-like exercise regimen. We only need to take small steps toward better health. We need only to begin.

eat well

Food is the fuel that makes our engine go. We wouldn't fill our car with any old type of fuel and expect it to run properly, so

Don't think of healthy eating in terms of *denying* yourself; think in terms of *nurturing* yourself. Look at what you can *add* to your diet instead of what you need to take away.

why would we assume we could do the same with our bodies? We should treat our body with respect and give it what it needs to function properly, like choosing good, nutri-tious whole foods that will give us the energy we need, and eating regular meals to keep our body from sputtering out on us by midday.

There are seven steps that I think are important to follow for the healthiest eating lifestyle. Each step is easy to implement. Each step carries a great payoff.

my seven steps to healthy eating

1   Know what your body needs to be healthy
2   Choose seasonal, fresh, and organic foods whenever possible
3   Vary your choices
4   Eat regular meals
5   Replace bad habits with good ones
6   Eat consciously
7   Embrace the joy and celebration of food

step one: know what your body needs to be healthy

WHOLE FOODS

The best way to work toward your healthiest body is to eat whole foods—foods closest to their original state. Whole foods are unprocessed, which means they are not altered from what nature intended. Processed foods, on the other hand, are modified from their natural state for transportation, preservation, or flavor. Brown rice, for example, is unprocessed. It comes to us the way it is grown and harvested, while the more common white rice has been bleached, losing most of its nutrients in the process, so we miss out on its natural benefits.

If you really want to stay strong and healthy and benefit from the vitality that whole foods can bring, try selections from the following list of what I like to call Super Foods!

Asparagus—a good source of folic acid, vitamin C, beta-carotene, and fiber.

Beans—contain many important healing nutrients like fiber, potassium, folic acid, and magnesium. Easy to add—put them in a salad, make them into a spread like hummus, or turn them into soup.

Blackstrap molasses—two tablespoons have more potassium than a banana and as much as a glass of milk. Try it spread on whole-grain bread or use as a sweetener in sauces.

Brewer's yeast—a good source of some very healing vitamins and minerals, including chromium, potassium, folic acid, and vitamin B_6. Stir a tablespoon or two into orange juice or a blender drink.

Broccoli—high in vitamin C, beta-carotene, and calcium. Good preventive food choice.

Cantaloupe—high in beta-carotene, potassium, and vitamin C. Many ways to be enjoyed—with a scoop of cottage cheese in the middle, for example, or my favorite, with a sprinkle of salt or topped with prosciutto. Delicious for breakfast.

Carrots—no better source of beta-carotene. Try marinated carrots as an accompaniment to sandwiches. Add jam or ginger jelly to cooked carrots for a sweet glaze.

Dried apricots—a good source of beta-carotene, potassium, and fiber. Stew them and swirl through oatmeal or spread on a bagel.

Fat-free yogurt—especially high in calcium—can provide 450 milligrams in just one cup.

Flaxseed—a wonderful antioxidant with a great nutty flavor. It has a lot of omega-3 fatty acids, and can also be very high in lignans, which are reported to have anti-tumor properties. Also helpful in alleviating menopausal symptoms.

Greens—the darker, the better. Try spinach, romaine, escarole, and Swiss chard. Good calcium sources: mustard greens, turnip greens, collard greens, kale, and bok choy. Some greens are good steamed, or sautéed with garlic and balsamic vinegar or ginger and soy.

Nuts—yes, they are high in fat, but they are also a great source of fiber and minerals like copper and chromium. Good to eat one to two tablespoons a day regularly. Get a cereal that contains nuts, add nuts to a stir-fry, or add to a salad. I love snacking on raw almonds.

Oats—high in protein and a wonderful source of fiber. Drizzle hot oatmeal with maple syrup or sprinkle with berries.

Papaya—great source of vitamin C and beta-carotene.

Prunes—sometimes called *dried* plums, are loaded with potassium and fiber. Prune puree can be substituted for oil or butter in baking. Stuff prunes with sweetened ricotta cheese for a special treat. (Other dried fruits, including figs, apples, and peaches, are also high in fiber.)

Red pepper—high in vitamin C and beta-carotene. Add to stir-fry, marinara sauce, or salad.

Ricotta cheese—has about four times as much calcium as cottage cheese. You can make it into a flavored spread for bagels, muffins, and crackers, or to fill an egg-white omelet or pasta shells. Dilute it for a creamy pasta sauce.

Salmon—an excellent source of "good fats," omega-3s, which can decrease inflammation and clotting of the blood. Choose small portion sizes and minimize rich sauces to maximize benefits.

Soy—a popular protein which helps reduce the risk of breast cancer and decreases the severity of menopausal symptoms. For optimal benefits eat in conjunction with calcium-rich foods.

Sweet potatoes or yams—the redder the skin, the more beta-carotene. Great source of potassium. Bake for forty-five minutes to an hour in a 400-degree oven.

Wheat bran—an insoluble fiber, like a broom for your digestive system! Also high in potassium and vitamin B_6.

Wheat germ—great source of vitamin E, also high in magnesium and folic acid. Mix it into blender drinks or sprinkle over cereal and yogurt. Keep in the refrigerator.

YOU ARE AT GREATER RISK FOR OSTEOPOROSIS IF YOU

- *are a postmenopausal Caucasian woman*

- *didn't get enough calcium during your childhood*

- *don't exercise regularly*

- *drink alcohol excessively*

- *have a petite frame*

- *are underweight*

- *are an athlete, former athlete, or someone who has exercised strenuously*

what we need every day

Whole foods—and Super Foods!—are an essential source of vitamins, minerals, proteins, carbohydrates, and fats. But what do we need to consume, in what quantities, and in what combination? How should we "budget" our nutrition? Read on . . .

GETTING WHAT WE NEED EVERY DAY

WHAT WE NEED	HOW MUCH	BEST FOOD SOURCES
Calcium	1,000–1,500 milligrams	Part skim mozzarella cheese, 1 cup (965 mg)
		Skim milk, 1 cup (304 mg)
		Fortified orange juice, 1 cup (300 mg)
		Nonfat yogurt, 1 cup (451 mg)
Vitamin A	4,000–5,000 International Units	Sweet potatoes, 1 cup (2,488 IU)
		Butternut squash, 1 cup (1,428 IU)
		Carrots, 1 cup (2,025 IU)
Vitamin B_6	2 milligrams	Banana, medium size (.7 mg)
		Red peppers, 1 cup (.4 mg)
		Brown rice, 1 cup cooked (.3 mg)
Vitamin C	60–75 milligrams	Orange, medium size (69 mg)
		Strawberries, 1 cup (86.2 mg)
		Red cabbage, 1 cup (50 mg)

WHAT WE NEED	HOW MUCH	BEST FOOD SOURCES
Vitamin D	400–600 International Units	Fortified skim milk, 1 cup (100 IU)
Vitamin E	22–30 International Units	Wheat germ, toasted, 1/4 cup (5.1 IU)
		Peanut butter, 2 tbs (4.8 IU)
		Sunflower seeds, 1 oz (21 IU)
Folate (folic acid)	400 micrograms	Chickpeas, 1 cup cooked (282 mcg)
		Pinto beans, 1 cup cooked (294 mcg)
		Asparagus, 1 cup cooked (131 mcg)
Fiber	25–30 grams	Lentils, 1 cup cooked (16 gm)
		Bran cereal, 1 cup (25 gm)
		Raisins, 1/2 cup (6.3 gm)
		Figs, 1/2 cup dried (12 gm)
		Baked potato with skin, medium size (7 gm)
		Pinto beans, 1/2 cup (9.8 gm)

WHAT WE NEED	HOW MUCH	BEST FOOD SOURCES
Iron	10 mg	Beef, liver, 3 oz (7.5 mg)
		Kidney beans, 1/2 cup (3.0 mg)
		Spinach, 1/2 cup (2.0 mg)
Omega-3 Fatty Acids	1.1 grams	Atlantic salmon, 4 oz (3 gm)
		Rainbow trout, 4 oz (2.3 gm)
		White tuna, canned and drained, 3.7 oz (2.6 gm)
		Walnuts, 3 tbs (1.1 gm)
		Flaxseed oil, 1 tbs (7.6 gm)
Omega-6 Fatty Acids	12 grams	Walnuts, 3 tbs (15 gm)
		Safflower oil, 1 tbs (13 gm)
		Pine nuts, 3 tbs (13 gm)

CALCIUM

Developing strong bones is important to our overall health at *every* age. Bone strength peaks between the ages of twenty-five and thirty, but many women begin to lose bone mass as early as their thirties. That's why it's important to eat enough calcium-rich foods to make up for the natural depletion caused by the aging process. When the level of calcium in our blood is low, our body "borrows" calcium from our bones. Over time, this can result in a lower bone

Eliminate soft drinks, including diet sodas. Not only are they empty calories, they actually leach calcium from our bones!

GOT CALCIUM? A CAUTIONARY TALE

What woman worried about her bones in her twenties? I know I didn't. And yet, the more I learn about bones at midlife, the more I find myself wishing that I had. I'm not alone.

Some time ago, my friend Regina accompanied her mother to her doctor's office for a bone density scan. While waiting, she decided she would also take the test to show support for her mother. A triathlete in her middle thirties, Regina was in great shape and thought she didn't really need the test. So imagine her shock when she got the results of the fifteen-minute scan and learned that she had the bone density of a sixty-five-year-old woman!

Regina was a competitive swimmer who had been swimming since she was a child. Even though she was getting plenty of physical exercise, she was participating in a *non-weight-bearing sport,* one that did not help build her bones. Regina was fortunate that she discovered her low bone density in time to make changes. Now she is careful to choose calcium-rich foods and avoid those that leach calcium from her bones, such as coffee and colas. Thankfully, as a result of her efforts, her bone density has increased and according to her latest bone scan, Regina shows results much *younger* than her age.

mass, which in turn can result in osteoporosis. Osteoporosis is a debilitating disease that causes our bones to become brittle and fragile, leading to potentially fatal falls and fractures. With advanced cases of osteoporosis, our bones literally cannot support us any longer.

Five ways we can protect ourselves from osteoporosis:

1   Increase the amount of calcium in our diet

2   Exercise regularly—weight-bearing

3   Reduce the amount of salt we take in

4   Drink fewer alcoholic beverages

5   Quit smoking

Sources of Calcium: Milk, tofu, soybeans, nonfat yogurt, salmon, sardines, scallops, spinach, kale, collard greens, bok choy, broccoli, broccoli rabe, beans, peas, dried figs, bananas, calcium-fortified orange juice, and citrus fruits.

COMPLEX CARBOHYDRATES

I think that carbs are getting a bum rap. They're the first things we're told to avoid in so many of the fad diets, but our bodies need them to keep us energized. The question is, *what kind?* "Simple" carbs, found in sugar and sweets, give us a "sugar high," a quick burst of energy that doesn't stay with us. "Complex" carbs also give us energy, but stay with us for the long haul. So choose the complex carbs, found in nonstarchy vegetables and whole-grain foods. They contain more fiber, so our body absorbs these carbohydrates at a slower rate, sustaining us longer with a steady flow of energy. Over the length of a demanding day, that's something we can count on.

We need to choose our carbohydrates carefully though, by balancing them proportionately with proteins and fats. When we do, the good news is that carbohydrates can actually help us *lose* weight.

I've had to figure out the best way to eliminate unnecessary carbs from my diet because I do love sugar. But if I get more of the healthier carbs, I can afford some sweets here and there. And we all need room to be "bad" once in a while!

Sources of Complex Carbohydrates: Legumes; nonstarchy vegetables, including leafy green ones; berries; apples; cherries; whole-grain foods.

FATS

We all know by now that we need to limit the amount of fat we eat, but we may not know that there's a difference in the *types* of fats we consume: healthy fats and unhealthy fats. What's the distinction? The healthy fats—polyunsaturated and monounsaturated—keep our skin and hair healthy, and our organs functioning properly. The unhealthy culprits—saturated fats—are the ones we need to avoid; they give us high cholesterol.

Healthy fats can be found in olives, olive and canola oil, nuts, and avocado. The omega-3 fats found in fatty fish, flaxseed oil, soy foods, walnuts, and pumpkin seeds are extremely healthy, as are the omega-6 oils found in nuts, egg yolks, organ meats, polyunsaturated vegetable oils, and plant seed oils such as evening primrose oil. The body needs both omega-3 and omega-6 oils, but since we can't produce these oils naturally, we need to get them from food. Steer clear of the unhealthy fats such as the saturated fats found in animal fats and full-fat dairy, and also from trans fat, which can be found in margarine and vegetable shortening.

Fat-free products add more sugar to compensate for flavor lost when the fat is removed—so when we eat fat-free, we're actually eating *more* calories!

Choose the "good guys." Steam or bake your food, instead of frying, and save the slice of pizza or pat of butter for special occasions. These small changes will make a noticeable difference in how your body looks and feels.

SOURCES OF FAT—THE HEALTHY ONES

POLYUNSATURATED	MONOUNSATURATED
Health Benefits: Reduces "bad" (LDL) cholesterol and risk of heart disease.	Health Benefits: Increases "good" (HDL) cholesterol, boosts the immune system, and reduces risk of heart disease and certain types of cancer.
<ul><li>grains</li><li>vegetables</li><li>safflower, sunflower, corn, and soybean oils</li><li>fatty fish, such as salmon and mackerel</li><li>flaxseeds</li></ul>	<ul><li>olive, peanut, and canola oils</li><li>nuts such as almonds, walnuts, cashews, and pecans</li><li>avocados</li></ul>

FIBER

Fiber keeps our whole system moving, literally. It keeps us regular, which makes our body feel better and our skin look great. Not to mention what it does for our mood.

Fiber lowers our cholesterol and our risk for colon cancer and heart disease. Fiber also slows digestion, giving us more nutrients over a longer period of time. It's low in carbohydrates and fat, helping us maintain a healthy weight. Fiber also makes us feel full, so we are less likely to overeat.

Sources of Fiber: Whole grains; fruits and vegetables, especially raspberries, spinach, sweet potato, and avocado; legumes (put cold lentils in a salad for a delicious way to get extra fiber; also split peas, navy beans, and chickpeas); and nuts, but go easy on portions—nuts do contain a lot of fat and calories.

FOLIC ACID

Folic acid helps strengthen the immune system, keeping us healthy and able to fight off any illnesses. It also fortifies our brain and nervous system.

Sources of Folic Acid: Chickpeas, pinto beans, asparagus, soybeans, spinach, seeds, and nuts. I like to toss sunflower and pumpkin seeds into a salad. (A handful of raw almonds is one of my favorite snacks.)

OMEGA-3

Ever since I've learned about the fabulous benefits of omega-3, I'm more excited about eating salmon—grilled or poached, hot or cold—I love it! Omega-3 fatty acids help keep our skin, hair, eyes, and nerves healthy, as well as our sweet heart. Omega-3 reduces our risk of heart disease, arthritis, and irritable bowel syndrome (IBS). These fatty acids regulate our blood pressure, enhance our immune system, unclog our arteries, and may even ease depression.

Sources of Omega-3: Cold-water fish, including salmon (my favorite), sardines, tuna (my second favorite), and herring; soy products; nuts and seeds, and nut oils; broccoli; beans; lettuce and spinach.

PHYTOCHEMICALS

Phytochemicals, found only in fruits and vegetables, boost immunity and health, lower our risk of chronic disease, and may even ward off cancer. It's amazing to me that we can have some health insurance in a delicious avocado or a juicy peach.

Fruits and vegetables also contain flavonoids—pigments that give them their color. They help keep our faithful heart

To get the most out of fruits and vegetables, choose the ones with the brightest colors—they have the most nutrients, especially the red and dark green ones.

pumping, minimize those hot flashes, and may help keep cataracts at bay. They are just what we need at midlife.

SOURCES OF PHYTOCHEMICALS

WHAT THEY ARE	WHY THEY'RE GOOD
Blueberries	High in antioxidants; antiaging; protect against cancer; and are thought to help memory
Strawberries and other red fruits	High in fiber, vitamin C, and potassium; lower cholesterol and risk of hypertension; protect against cancer
Cantaloupe, oranges, and other orange fruits	High in beta-carotene, folic acid, vitamin C, and antioxidants; protect vision; guard against heart disease, arthritis, diabetes, and cancer
Tomatoes and other red vegetables	Contain fiber and vitamin C; slow skin aging; protect against cancer
Cabbage, broccoli, Brussels sprouts, bok choy, mustard greens, and other leafy dark green vegetables	High in fiber, calcium, folic acid, and vitamin C; protect against heart disease and cancer
Sea kelp, seaweed	High in protein and omega-3; promote strong bones; boost metabolism
Leafy dark green vegetables, especially spinach	High in antioxidants; contain folic acid, iron, vitamins C and E, calcium and protein; neutralize free radicals; protect against cancer

PHYTOESTROGENS

Asians have known the secret of eating soy protein for centuries; now, in the U.S., we're learning more about how it can help us. Soy contains natural hormones, called phytoestrogens, which are rich in antioxidants, protecting us against all kinds of diseases, and slowing down the aging process.

I grind flaxseed in my coffee grinder and keep the powder in a container in the fridge. Whenever I can, I sprinkle some on my salad, oatmeal, dry cereal, or even yogurt.

In women, phytoestrogens also help regulate estrogen levels, making them a vital support for midlife. They reduce menopausal symptoms, such as hot flashes, and can help us with decreased sexual drive.

Sources of Phytoestrogens: Soybeans, tofu, soy milk, soy yogurt, apples, carrots, oats, plums, olives, sunflower seeds, potatoes, tea, coffee, and flaxseed.

PROTEIN

We all need energy! energy! energy! Not just for "keeping up," but for doing everything we want and now, at midlife, have the time to do. Protein converts easily to energy. It also helps us maintain our muscle mass and fight infection.

We often think of meat first as a protein source, but in fact the healthiest kind of protein comes from plants, not animals. Studies have shown that America's fifteen million vegetarians have lower cancer and hypertension rates than the general public. They also have decreased risk of heart disease, greater longevity, and an easier time managing their weight. All the more reason to get in those vegetables.

We should limit the amount of meat we eat, because animal protein contains more of the "bad" fats, is high in cholesterol, and is harder for our body to digest. If your choice is toward meat and poultry, try to choose those that have been raised without suffering; free-range chicken and beef, and even kosher meat and organic eggs. It's a better choice, both nutritionally and ethically. And don't forget fish. It is a great alternative to meat and poultry, and a wonderful source of protein.

Sources of Protein

PLANT-BASED PROTEIN Soy products, legumes, nuts and seeds, "wheat meats" (such as vegi-burgers, seitan burgers, and soy dogs), whole grains, and rice-based products. Boca Foods make wonderful meatless burgers and sausages. I heartily recommend them (see Resource Guide).

ANIMAL-BASED PROTEIN Dairy products, fish, lean beef and pork, skinless chicken, and turkey.

H$_2$OH!

Keep a bottle of water near you throughout the day.

Whenever you pass a water fountain, stop for a few sips. Sipping water all day keeps us hydrated and curbs snack attacks (sometimes pangs of hunger are our body's signal for more water).

Look for "natural" or "pure" spring water rather than "purified" water, which is often city water that has been distilled to remove contaminants.

Remember that any drink with caffeine is a diuretic that will deplete your body of water. Alcohol will also dehydrate the body. If you drink coffee, tea, or soda, add an *extra* glass of water each time to replace the water that they take out of your body.

Watch out for sports drinks too. They can contain a lot of sugar and sodium and add unwanted calories.

Try to drink at least eight glasses of water a day, more if you are very active.

Experiment with different bottled waters; they have beneficial trace elements and different flavors—find one you like.

Put a drop of natural syrup, mint, lemon, lime, or orange in your water—vary with your favorite flavorings.

WATER

I reach for water to manage that four o'clock energy dip, and I've found that drinking a big glass of water, instead of coffee, actually gives me a lift.

Water in the morning, water in the evening—at our bedside table, on our desk, in our tote—we simply can't afford to skip it. We need to replace our fluids constantly because we lose about two to three quarts every day. Water allows us to absorb more nutrients, regulate our temperature, cushion our joints, and flush toxins from our system. Even a little dehydration can slow us down. When we're just slightly dehydrated we get sluggish, our energy levels dip, and our concentration wavers. Drinking water helps perk us up almost immediately. Don't wait to "catch up" on water—by the time we actually feel thirsty, we are already dehydrated. So keep the H_2O flowing!

step two: choose seasonal, fresh, and organic foods whenever possible

I like to eat the freshest foods possible. It just makes sense that food eaten closer to the time it has been picked will contain more vitality. The more vitality in food, the more energy it gives us, paying off in better health, younger looks, and longer life—that's a pretty good deal.

My first choice is to buy organic—foods produced without chemicals—whenever I can. I'm pleased to say that it's a lot easier than it used to be to find and afford organic foods. Today, there are organic urban gardens and cooperatives in the biggest cities, and supermarkets across the country carry organic produce. I like the national chain Whole Foods Market. It really is a garden of earthly delights. I never have a problem finding what I want, and the food is always fresh. But you can ask your local grocer to carry your favorite organic foods—breads, yogurt, greens, veggies, and fruit— chances are he will happily accommodate you. There really is a big difference in the way that better-quality food makes us feel. And, many people, myself included, think that organic fruits and veggies also taste better.

Always read the labels to know what you're buying. Even "organic" is not always what it appears to be. Organic labels are divided into three categories:

- *100 percent Organic:* 100 percent of the packaged food has been grown organically.
- *Organic:* 95 percent of the packaged food has been grown organically.

- *Made with Organic:* Less than 70 percent of a product is made with organic ingredients.

The next-best thing to buying organic is getting fruits and vegetables in season, especially those grown by local farmers. If it's local, it's freshest. When foods are shipped long distances, the lag time between farm and fridge means vitamins lost. Eating produce at its peak is like adding another life force to our own. Farmers' markets are some of the best places to find the freshest food. I love to visit the local markets whenever I can, wherever I am. I particularly love the farmers' market in Santa Barbara—it's a pure joy. I talk to the growers and sample the bright, fresh fruits and vegetables that have just been picked. And I also make sure to sample the delicious jams and jellies too. To find a farmers' market in your area, visit the USDA's Web site (see Resource Guide).

As midlife women, both our buying power and role as the primary food shoppers for our households give us tremendous power to influence demand—and therefore supply and cost—of these items. With the wisdom of midlife, we can come to know that when we choose local and organic produce, not only are we getting the best for ourselves and our families, we're also doing a service for the land—choosing foods that are chemical-free and not putting those chemicals into the earth to pollute the streams and crops of our future. As mothers, grand-mothers, and people who care, we know that *how* food is grown affects not only us but also the generations to come.

step three: vary your choices

While I was taking classes at New York's Culinary Institute, Richard, my favorite teacher and chef, said that most of us have the *same* seven meals over and over again. For some of us, that number could be even less. If this is true, how can we manage to get all the different vitamins and minerals we need to stay healthy?

Varying our choices allows us to break our food boundaries, to become adventurous, and stay healthy.

There is an infinite variety of cuisines out there, just waiting for us to savor them: delicate mint salad tabbouleh from Lebanon; hearty bouillabaisse from France; tender edamame from Japan; spicy curries and cooling yogurt—*raita*—from India; the endlessly delicious variety of pastas from Italy; tasty steamed Chinese dumplings; and hot Caribbean dishes. Not only do these foods satisfy our craving for exotic flavors, but also, more importantly, they bring much-needed vitamins and minerals into our diet.

Variety in food *is* the spice of life. It really does keep us from being bored, and is a source of joy and whimsy. At midlife, we need to keep our senses active; for some of us, aging can diminish our senses, including taste and smell. I love to experiment with flavors: a swath of olive oil, some sea salt, and a little squeeze of lemon on grilled fish; hot wasabi peas as a snack; minced rosemary or chopped cilantro in a soup; basil or a little sesame oil in a salad; cayenne pepper in a pasta dish. Once you discover new foods, and also how herbs and spices can enhance natural flavors, you'll experiment on your own.

LIFE IS THE VARIETY OF SPICE—SOME FAVORITES

Herbs can add life to your meals—and they may also add years to your life. According to researchers at the U.S. Department of Agriculture, herbs such as oregano and rosemary can actually help the body fight cancer. Fresh oregano, for example, has forty-two times the antioxidant power of apples!

VINEGARS	HERBS	SPICES	SWEET FLAVORS
Balsamic	Rosemary	Jalapeño peppers	Barley malt
Rice	Thyme	Cayenne peppers	Honey
Mirin	Basil	Dijon mustard	Rice syrup
Umeboshi (a Japanese vinegar made from salted, pickled plums with a tangy flavor)	Tarragon	Chilies	Maple syrup
	Parsley	Curry	Apple butter
	Mint		
	Oregano		
	Cilantro		

step four: eat regular meals

Skipping meals is not a good way to lose weight. When we go without food we actually signal to our body that we are in starvation mode, and, in a panic, our body responds by holding on to our stored energy sources—our fat. Our body doesn't know when—or if—we're ever going to eat again, so it hoards what's available, storing it on our hips, tummies, and thighs. (This is a survival instinct from our earliest cavewoman days—long before takeout—when we didn't know if our foraging mates would be hauling anything home for dinner.) So I love to remind women that to lose weight, we need to eat, and to eat regularly. That way we don't send panic signals to our bodies, and we can *e-e-ease* them into shape.

When we don't feed our body and it automatically goes into survival mode, it does the opposite of what we want—storing our fat and basically "eating" our muscle. Skipping meals also means we are likely to suffer from decreased energy, mood swings, and irritability.

We all have difficulty eating regularly, because of lack of time, stress, or our appetite fluctuations. One strategy to get around the three-square-meals-a-day ideal is to eat several smaller meals a day. Eating smaller meals helps us keep our energy high. This is much healthier than eating three large meals a day, and certainly smarter than skipping them.

step five: replace bad habits with good ones

Habits develop over time and eventually become a way of life. At midlife, we recognize that we need to let go of habits that don't support us and replace them with habits that do.

We are now able to make more informed choices to influence our future. We are motivated more than ever to develop good habits because we have the perspective to see the cause and effect between our lifestyle and our health more clearly.

It took years for our habits to become second nature for us, and it will take some patience and discipline to exchange bad habits for good ones. For instance, I *love* coffee. It's my weakness. I love coffee flavor in everything: yogurt, chocolate, ice cream. What would life be without a cappuccino! But I do realize coffee has its drawbacks.

Coffee is an appetite suppressant; it interferes with our ability to recognize when we are hungry, so we're not always in touch with what our body needs, or what it is trying to tell us. It's vital to our health that we learn to recognize when we're hungry—*and* when we're full—and when we're tired. When we override these signals, not only do we "disconnect" from our body, we put a strain on it. Coffee stresses our adrenals, weakens our immune system, and dehydrates us—not to mention giving us the jitters. Did you know that caffeine even draws water *from* our body? And, we know by now the problems that arise when we don't get enough water.

By replacing coffee with green tea, we break a bad habit by exchanging it for a better one. We still have the "coffee break," but with a much more nurturing drink that has many added bonuses. Green tea boosts our metabolism, increases the amount of energy our body burns, and offers us protection against heart disease, high cholesterol, high blood pressure, cancer, and osteoporosis and gives us a powerful source of antioxidants. I try alternating my coffee with a steaming cup of green tea. Guayakí Yerba Maté is another healthy alternative to coffee. A powerful rejuvenating beverage grown in the rain forest, it's healthy and tasty (see Resource Guide).

A box of tea won't do you any good if it's collecting dust on the shelf, so experiment with your teas and find what suits you best. To make a cup of tea really special, you might like to try adding a spoonful of French Deluxe Vanilla Powder (available from The Coffee Bean and Tea Leaf; see Resource Guide). It makes regular tea taste oh so rich. And if you find, as I do, that you like everything sweet, try sweetening your tea with SteviaTabs Stevia Extract (see Resource Guide). It's a safe and tasty way to sweeten your tea—and it's also a nutrient.

strategies for changing bad to better

- Don't skip breakfast—it keeps your energy high all day, so you'll be less likely to indulge "bad" cravings.

- Never shop for food on an empty stomach.

- Carry a shopping list of healthy foods to the supermarket. If you don't have "bad" things in your house, you won't eat them.

- Use a smaller serving plate as a dinner plate.

- Always carry healthy snacks with you to catch a blood-sugar dive before it drives you to eat anything sugary.

- Prepare key ingredients for a week's worth of meals on Sunday. Turn on some great upbeat music and chop, mince, and dice. Keep the ingredients in Tupperware containers. It will be much easier for you to cook fresh food throughout the week if you've saved time on the preparation.

- Make lunch the main meal of your day; your metabolism slows down at night, making it more likely you'll gain weight from big dinners, especially big, late dinners.

- Schedule snacks the same as you would your breakfast and dinner, especially for the four o'clock energy lag.

- You stop cravings when you eat fresh, whole foods, because you're getting *all* your nutrients.

- Before I make or order a meal, I try to review what I have already eaten that day. I make a game of it. Did I get enough protein or vegetables? (Sometimes I realize I haven't had any fruit in several days.) This way, I'm more aware of what I need to give my body on a continuing basis.

- If you really have to have that piece of cake, don't deny yourself—just have half, and eat it *very* slowly. If you deny yourself, you'll eventually end up eating the *whole* cake!

GOOD HABITS EXCHANGED FOR BAD

EMBRACE	AVOID (AS MUCH AS POSSIBLE)
Whole foods	Processed foods
1% or 2% milk	Whole milk
Olive oil	Oils with high saturated fats, such as coconut, palm kernel, peanut, and margarine
Fatty fish	Red meat
Baked, grilled, or steamed	Fried
Green or black tea	Coffee
Balsamic vinegar and olive oil	Salad dressings made with hydrogenated oils, soybean oils, egg yolks, and creams

In Eastern philosophy, food is considered as God, and all food is treated with that kind of respect. As wise women, we want to embrace conscious eating as an essential part of both honoring our body *and* nurturing our spirit.

step six: eat consciously

Eating consciously is about knowing what our body needs to be healthy. Equally important is being *aware* of what you are eating.

What do I mean by being aware of what you eat? Well, consider my girlfriend Colleen. She's a vivacious woman, an enthusiastic person who just loves life. She also loves to eat and at times struggles with her weight. Once, while we were having dinner, she was so intent on talking to me that she never once really looked down at her plate. Colleen is very animated, and she talked so quickly, spilling out her story, that there wasn't a pause between mouthfuls. At the end of the meal, I noticed her completely empty plate and said to her, "Don't look down at your plate and tell me what you just had for dinner." She couldn't answer! She had been so wrapped up in her story that she was unconscious as she ate and didn't remember what she had eaten. Then how could her food have properly nourished her?

For me, eating begins with the eyes. If we can't take a moment to really see and appreciate what is on our plate, to gracefully receive food first through our eyes, then how can we receive all of its goodness properly into our body? Eating well is being aware of the food in front of us and knowing we've made the best choices for our health. Then we've already made an agreement with what is on our plate. We are in harmony; we have a relationship, a receptive relationship, with the food that is about to nourish us. We could take this a step further. When we eat, we are, in effect, exchanging one life form to support another. The food we eat is being offered up for our survival. Knowing this, we want to honor the sacrifice that has been made to support us.

Conscious eating also means really *tasting* what we're eating, by chewing it thoroughly, at least twenty-five times, allowing more of the nutrients to be broken down in our mouth instead of in our digestive system. This way our food can fully "feed" us. This takes a tremendous strain off our internal organs, and gives us the full value of the nutrients in our food. It also makes digestion much easier and is great for weight control, because the essential nutrients are more thoroughly absorbed.

Unconscious eating shows itself in a myriad of ways. Perhaps we keep jumping from one diet to another. Or we skip meals. Or maybe we plop ourself in front of the television, with a box of cookies in one hand and a bag of chips in the other. Fast food, junk food, snacks, and cookies may have worked with the "who cares" or "whatever" unconscious lifestyle of our younger years, but our nutritional needs at midlife are different, and we are smarter now. If we have continued eating unconsciously in this way, by midlife our reserves are nearing depletion. We can't expect to keep going without changing our old bad habits.

Eating consciously is the *best* way we can eat well. Know that every time you make a conscious, positive choice to honor your body with healthy food, you are honoring your life. Today I choose foods that are nutritious, but I still give myself the freedom to slip in a cookie from time to time, a muffin, or a piece of great cake (okay, maybe *half* a piece of cake . . .).

step seven: embrace the joy and celebration of food

The smells, the sounds, the taste of foods, and the love we show our families as we share meals, all come together around the table. Mealtime is our opportunity to combine the magic of food with our love and connection to family and friends.

Even before we join together to share a delicious meal, the aroma of cooking works on a subtle, sensual level to convey to us a sense of well-being. And how we prepare our food also influences how we will receive it. I feel it is important to cook and serve food with loving thoughts. As we cook, the combination of the Shakti—"life force"—in food and our own loving energy make our home come alive.

While writing this book I stayed part of the time in a house just south of Provence. The simple stucco-and-terra-cotta cottage and its gardens had been neglected by an absent owner and indifferent renters and clearly hadn't been loved enough. Yet, the combined energy of a devoted cook and loving guests rejuvenated our little abode. As a delicious lunch was prepared, I noticed an amazing transformation take place.

When Pascal, the chef, commanded the kitchen, the individual aromas of all the different ingredients gently wafted throughout the house, making it feel homey. We were uplifted by each new smell, one after the other, as he went about preparing the meal: first olive oil and garlic, then basil, onion, tomato, mushrooms, and ginger, followed by sugar being caramelized and apples baking—and then the heavenly blend they created together!

The sounds of the meal being created added to our sense of well-being. As we worked, we heard the intermittent sizzle of vegetables as they hit the pan, the crackle of fresh fish sautéing, the gentle slap of lettuce against the ceramic salad bowl. Even the voices engaged in intense food preparation fed our anticipation of the meal, conveying a feeling of being taken care of. Knowing we were about to be so lovingly nourished, we finally felt we had made our house a home.

All the aspects of food have a transformational effect when we treat them with great respect. By recognizing that food sustains all life on the planet, it takes on a blessed aspect. The holy Hindu Upanishad texts praise the sacred nature of food by saying, "All creatures that dwell on earth are born of food and live through food."

The great teacher Swami Chidvilasananda wrote in *The Yoga of Discipline:*

Food is the healing herb that nourishes all.
Whoever worships (God) as food wants for nothing.

When we take time to sit together and share a deliciously prepared meal, we express our love and gratitude not only for what is on our plate, but also for one another. That's why saying a prayer before a meal is such a poignant moment of pause. When we honor what is in front of us, we enhance our experience; we realize and pay tribute to all the efforts it took to bring the meal before us; the fisherman who netted the day's catch, the fruits and vegetables that offered themselves to us, the trees and ground that nurtured them, the farmer who tended them, the helpers who sorted, the drivers who brought the food to market, the chef, the guests with whom we share our meal—all deserve our gratitude. When we glimpse the magnitude of a single meal, realizing all that it took to bring it to our table, gratitude naturally swells. In that instant we have turned an everyday act into an extraordinary moment.

There is nothing that bonds us more than coming together and sharing a memorable meal. I recall so many vivid moments at my French friend Elisabeth's magical farm in St. Tropez. Her home is so alive, the food delicious, the atmosphere transformative; people literally fight to come there!

Cooking done with care is an act of love.

—CRAIG CLAIBORNE

Our day starts with the preparation for the lunch and dinner to come. Elisabeth and I hit the market early. First we visit Christine, the *poissonnière* (fish seller), who proudly displays the morning's catch. She recommends a *loup de mer*—a sea bass—and expertly stuffs the center with fresh fennel. Then, with a big grin, she hands it over to us, accompanied by a tidbit of local gossip.

Next, the *fromagerie*—the cheese shop. As you walk into the shop, the pungent smells of cheese instantly wake you up. The owner laughs heartily as he proudly shows us the full range of his cheeses, from mild to strong; we taste them and debate over which ones the guests will savor at dinner. Then, and only then, are we ready for the parade of colors that strikes us as we descend on the open fruit and vegetable market.

Knowing all the vendors by name, we weave our way through the stalls. The vibrant red of the peppers and radishes, the cooling greens of the zucchini and haricots verts, the sweet scent of ripe melons in the air! The array of produce is like musical notes that play over our senses. Finally, our arms filled to the brim with our bounty, anticipation of the impending meal dancing in our head, we zoom home.

Now the cooking begins. Suddenly the farm is transformed. First, the calm, quiet peeling of the vegetables; as we sit under the shade of the pine trees, rows of vineyards stretch out before us. We catch up on the day's events while we make the hors d'oeuvres. Then the main course; as we prepare the fish, the fragrance starts to wend its way out of the kitchen and into the other rooms. The table is set, dancing with the joyous colors of Provence. Fresh-cut, fat, "oomphy" pink and yellow roses dot the table. The candles are lit. In an hour or so, the meal is ready. The stage is now set; we await the players. Now don't you wish you were with us?

I find that in the slow disintegration of the family unit, as many of us move farther and farther away from each other, we are losing the ritual of the family union over a meal. With all our day-to-day pressures, we've opted for convenience over tradition, and in doing so, we have lost not only an opportunity to come together and strengthen our ties with family and friends, we have also lost that sense of excitement and wonder that makes every meal a celebration. When I spend time in France and Italy, I find myself immersed again and again in the celebration of food that has not been forgotten, as we embrace the joyous tradition of life around the family table.

I'm always amazed how coming together around a bountiful and beautiful table puts people in an expansive, jovial mood; that is when people are at their best, and magic starts to happen. In Europe, the generations still come together, *every day,* just like the old days, and life is celebrated, along with food. We, too, can create more opportunities to make the family table a magic experience.

exercise

Regular exercise is vital to honoring your body. And the key word here is *regular.* You cannot have a strong, healthy body without regular activity. The good news is that simply by exercising thirty minutes at least three times a week, you can improve your health, reduce body fat, fight disease, and relieve depression, tension, and stress. The benefits are endless.

Need further convincing? Consider this: According to the Centers for Disease Control and Prevention (CDC) some 60 percent of the U.S. population is overweight. And 250,000 to 300,000 deaths are attributed to inactivity every year. So listen to what the doctor says and try to fit in at least one half hour of low-intensity exercise three times a week.

> *To keep the body in good health is a duty.*
> —BUDDHA

Even a small amount of exercise can help you to greatly reduce your risk of heart disease. Don't wait until you have a health issue. Exercise now to prevent one.

why now?

Midlife women have witnessed a parade of exercise fads and diets. We've lived through the low-fat, low-carb, high-protein, no-sugar, all-fruit, all-vegetable, fasting, and starvation diets. We've been high-impact, low-impact, and no-impact, and at times have tried to make our bodies conform to someone else's ideal. It is time, once and for all, to learn to love our bodies as our own ideal, and to accept our own personal, healthy body shape as it truly is. And that means not measuring it against the impossible. There are as many beautiful body types around as there are people. Why do we all need to look alike? There are so many kinds of beauty, and the most important is *healthy* beauty. And that is within the reach of most of us.

KEEP MOVING AND . . .

- *Improve Your Outlook on Life:* **Regular exercise can significantly improve mental outlook and help keep depression at bay.**

- *Build Muscle:* **Our bodies burn an extra fifty calories a day for each pound of muscle gained. (For those who are interested, that means a "free" cookie!) Muscle also protects our bones.**

- *Maintain a Healthy Weight:* **Regular exercise has been proven to help long-term weight loss. Good news for the 60 percent of American adults who are overweight.**

- *Build Stronger Bones:* **Roughly one-third of women over age sixty-five will suffer a bone fracture due to osteoporosis. Weight-bearing activities create strong bones, protecting against fractures.**

- *Lower Your Risk of Heart Disease:* **Almost half a million women die of heart disease every year; more women's deaths than from cancer and diabetes combined. Exercising three times a week for only *thirty minutes* reduces this risk.**

Exercise is the key to having the best body we can. Not only does exercise help us to become strong and fit, no matter what our body type, but it encourages us to admire our body's capacity to do things that we thought were beyond us. My friend Michele has a beautiful body. It's not a photo model's body (thank goodness); it's more like the *Venus de Milo*—voluptuous, curvy, and feminine. (I think she would like that analogy, as she often laughs, "Why am I always the example of the chubby friend?") Michele has always been frustrated by exercising. She says that she is "not a *normal* exercise person." She tried regular gym workouts, Pilates, yoga, running clinics, and a few training sessions, but she always ended up bored and dissatisfied by the routines. None of the traditional methods held her interest. They made her feel good for a while, but they didn't excite her. In fact, they actually had a debilitating effect. Her frustration with her exercise routines led her to eat more and more, and as a result she became lethargic. Her body was in constant pain from lack of activity and accumulated stress, creating a vicious cycle that resulted in a lot of unhappiness. One day, out of sheer frustration, Michele tried something truly exotic: Wing Chun. A meditation in motion, Wing Chun is a martial art that teaches self-defense. It uses the energy of the obstacle with the minimum of effort, yet the practitioner remains centered and relaxed. Michele had found her niche! She had finally discovered an exercise that was in keeping with her own warrior spirit. It's been a year now since Michele started her classes and she rarely misses one. She loves it. It makes her feel alive. She has more energy, is mentally stimulated, has a tremendous feeling of well-being, and is able to apply the techniques she has learned in class to her day-to-day problems. What's more, Michele has discovered she now admires her body and all the amazing things it can do. She has learned to accept her own body type and has discovered the newfound power it has. Now Michele loves her warrior-like Venus de Milo body.

You too must not forget what a miracle your body is. At midlife, with the wisdom you now have, you need to see where the truth is and to—at last—make your body your own. Even if you have body issues (and I'll wager that there are few who haven't) you can finally, at midlife, learn to love your own body and treat it with respect.

the adventure of exercise

Many of us may find that midlife offers the freedom to attempt something we've never done before. We may have more time on our hands now, feel the need to realize a long-submerged dream for adventure, or feel we just *finally* want to get into shape. We have gone through many kinds of exercise over our life so far and we either need to be challenged more, like my friend Michele, or to find a way to work out that is more specific for our present needs. Be daring. Shake it up! Try canoeing or scuba diving or sailing. Take a fencing class. Experiment with the myriad forms of dance, or experience the simple, childlike joy of riding a bike again. I know one woman who went skiing for the very first time when she was in her fifties. Now she's past sixty, still skiing, still loving it. Don't think that you have to be a daredevil, though. Do what feels right for you.

For those of you who feel they have failed at exercise attempts, take heart. It's important to remember that research shows us that it takes about *eight weeks* to break a habit, no matter what that habit might be. So be patient with yourself and just keep on moving. And make it fun. Ten minutes here and there do add up. It's all cumulative. Don't give up. As Michele discovered, there is always a routine out there for you. You may need variety. You may need a couple of sessions with a trainer to get you started. You may need the encouragement of exercising with a friend or a group to keep you going. That's fine. If working out with others will help keep you committed, then that's what you should do. Find out what motivates you and follow through. But whatever you do, don't forget the willpower element. Willpower is an important factor in exercising. And we all need a dose of it. You have to make a commitment and you

Move your body. And make sure to have fun doing it!

The secrets to keeping up an exercise routine are:

1   *Weave it into your life on a regular basis.*

2   *Vary the routine so you don't burn out.*

3   *Find activities that you enjoy so you look forward to them.*

4   *Sneak exercise into your day whenever—and wherever—you can.*

have to have a goal. There will be moments when you won't feel like it. But aren't you just a little tired of saying "someday" about your exercise routine? Your someday can be today, if you choose. Your body will thank you for it in so many ways. Besides keeping you flexible, strong, and lean, exercise releases endorphins, which give you the great feeling that life is wonderful! What better motivator do you need?

Remember: Exercise isn't something that takes place just at the gym. Sometimes it's just too hard to squeeze a full workout into our already busy schedule or too hard to confront the idea of being "squeezed" into a leotard. Not to worry. Just look for the opportunities to move your body. They are there for you all day long; from side bends as you brush your teeth to walking around a soccer field at halftime if you are watching a game. When you slip exercise in during the day, there's a delicious feeling of "cheating" and the person who is winning is you.

While I'm washing the dishes, I often get my leg lifts in by tying a wide stretch elastic around my ankles. I sneak in a bit of exercise *and* my dishes sparkle! I've been known to squeeze in side bends when I'm waiting in line at the movies, and do tummy tighteners when I'm on the phone. The benefits of exercise really are incremental. Five minutes here and five minutes there can all add up to a fitter, more vital you.

easy ways to sneak movement into a busy day

- Take the stairs whenever you can.
- Park the car farther away from the store.
- Walk during your lunch hour.
- Make a standing invitation for a friend to take regular walks with you.
- Take a walk after dinner. In Italy, they call this a *passeggiata,* and the whole family goes along.
- Remember your childhood favorites: Fly a kite. Toss a Frisbee. Play kickball or softball with friends, children, or grandchildren.
- Make the next vacation an active one, such as downhill skiing or hiking, river rafting, canoeing, or kayaking.

- Ride a bike—one of my favorites—a great way to see the countryside.
- Get up from the sofa to change channels, instead of using the remote control—well, it's a start.

what exercise is best for you

Two types of exercise are particularly important for building and maintaining bone mass and density at midlife—weight-bearing exercises and resistance exercises. Weight-bearing exercises make your bones and muscles work *against* gravity. This group of exercises contains any activity in which your feet and legs bear your own weight, such as jogging, walking, stair climbing, dancing, and playing soccer. Resistance exercises involve moving objects (including our own body weight) to *create resistance* and strengthen our bones. Free weights, weight-training machines, and exercise bands are some ways to do resistance exercise. You should try to get in both resistance and weight-bearing exercise to keep your body strong and healthy. The good news is, there is no shortage of creative and interesting ways to get exercise. Here are a few to start you off:

Trampolines: A mini-trampoline is great fun! I use mine regularly. It offers the same benefits as aerobic sports and the best thing is that it brings out the kid in you.

Swimming: Swimming gives you a total workout, making it a great choice for all-over body tone. It strengthens your back muscles, all your major muscle groups, as well as your lungs and heart. Certain aquatic exercises create resistance, especially when you use paddles or fins.

Dance: Dance is more than aerobic exercise—it is a complete mind-body workout and an *amazing* way to de-stress from a challenging day. Get creative! Take lessons—salsa, ballroom, ballet, tap, jazz . . . how about belly dancing? Or just turn up the volume of your old ABBA CDs and dance around your living room!

Tai Chi: Tai chi is a slow, controlled series of poses, all weight-bearing movements. The poses require a concentration that is almost meditative. Tai chi makes you calmer and more centered while making you more physically fit.

Hiking: Hiking is an *active* form of relaxation, and a great weight-bearing exercise. It can be as challenging as you want and a great way to bond with family and friends.

Pilates: Pilates is a series of specific exercises using resistant springs, strengthening your muscles and keeping
you incredibly flexible. It's also very energizing.
Pilates focuses on the alignment of your body, which
improves your posture and balance.

Sometimes attitude can be the biggest impediment
to exercise—that old *can't-be-bothered* tape can play pretty
loudly sometimes. When that happens, I find that the easiest
way to recharge myself and to change my attitude is to go for
a walk. If I'm feeling a little sluggish, or perhaps I'm at a bit
of a loose end—not sure what I want to do and not in the
mood for the things I need to do—then I lace up my Nikes
and head to the park. I may not feel like it at the time, and it
may take a little discipline to get me going, but I have enough
experience to know how great I'll feel later,
and it's that thought that pushes me forward.
I'm always thankful that I made the effort. I
see the seasons change. I watch buds appear or
leaves turn golden and red. I breathe the fresh
air from the park. I watch people gaily greet
each other and bring their dogs together to joyfully play. I
delight in the various ways the park is used by everyone; the
bike riding, skating, the zoo, walking, violins and clowns, and

**The worst thing we
can do for our health
is nothing.**

puppeteers and acrobats. Everyone is alive and I am rejuvenated! Afterward, I have made a shift and everything looks just a little bit better. Then I am able to make more supportive choices in my life, choices that make me feel good about myself. After exercising, it's easy. I *naturally* reach for foods that are healthier, instead of the quick-fix candy bar or sticky bun. And, the nutritious foods I do eat give me the energy I need for the rest of my day, making me feel *even better.* It all starts with just a bit of exercise. The old adage "Use it or lose it" couldn't be truer.

get strong, stay strong

I can't emphasize strongly enough how important it is to strengthen our bones by exercising properly and eating well. The fact is if we want our bones to continue to support us throughout our lives, then we must support them. Right now.

Some women may think that taking care of our bones is only necessary in our old age. In fact, developing strong bones is important to our overall health at *every* age. Our bone strength peaks between the ages of twenty-five and thirty, and many women have already started to lose bone mass by their late thirties. Don't wait another day to start thinking about the health of your bones.

Since osteoporosis tends to run in families, some women

may be at higher risk than others. Certain prescription drugs can also increase the loss of bone density, especially steroid drugs, anticonvulsants, Valium, and Ativan. But take heart—there is still much we can do to prevent osteoporosis. Our primary defense is being conscientious about what we eat. Our level of bone strength is determined in our teens, and it's what we do or don't do after that that strengthens or diminishes our bones.

A recent study found that Okinawan women had stronger bones and a lower risk of osteoporosis even though their diets contained less calcium than those of American women. Because their diets are so high in soy products, they are able to use the calcium they are receiving more efficiently. As a result, the Okinawan women who ate the most soy had the densest bones. Many researchers think that isoflavones, estrogen-like compounds found in soy products, are the source of soy's benefits because they help our bones absorb calcium.

Women have less bone mass than men to begin with, so we have to be more vigilant. Roughly one in three women over the age of sixty-five suffers an osteoporosis-related fracture. Don't think that a bone fracture is something a doctor can easily mend. The sobering fact is that fractures caused by osteoporosis—literally, a loss of bone mass—*are a result of bone shattering*, making bones impossible to mend with a cast. But combining exercise with a regimen of vitamin D and calcium supplements can decrease your risk of fractures by 30 percent.

Just in case we didn't already have enough reasons to increase our calcium intake, we also know that calcium not only builds stronger bones but also helps keep weight off, protects our hearts, lowers our blood pressure, eases pre-menstrual symptoms, keeps our teeth healthy, and reduces our risk of stroke. A recent study from the Harvard Nurses' Health Study even found that low calcium intake was associated with increased risk of stroke in midlife women. It's enough to make you run for the cottage cheese—low-fat, of course!

rest

We know that we need to get enough rest, but many of us still tax our bodies to exhaustion with all we try to fit into a day. We never mean to, but somehow when it comes to sleep we find that it's just too easy to cheat ourselves. And that's what we do when we don't get enough sleep—we *cheat* ourselves. When we deny ourselves a good night's sleep we rob ourselves of the chance to repair our bodies and our minds. What a shame that is.

Never underestimate the immediate and restorative power of a good night's sleep (or even a stolen nap in the afternoon), and the effect it can have on our health and sense of well-being. We all need the proper amount of rest, especially by the time we reach midlife when we've experienced a lifetime of the challenges and frustrations of trying to make up for lost sleep.

Here's a wake-up call: According to *The Promise of Sleep*, getting enough sleep is one of the most significant forecasters of how long you will live!

Sleep difficulties, primarily caused by stress and worry, can increase gradually after age thirty-five, even among the healthiest of us. Our sleeping patterns can also be disturbed by menopausal symptoms: hot flashes may wake us in the middle of the night, and sleep deprivation can be excruciating, not only to our minds, but also to our depleted bodies. Losing sleep can cause moodiness and depression, make us more susceptible to infection, interfere with memory, and lead to unhealthy eating habits and weight gain. Because sleeping gives our body a chance to replace aging or dead skin cells, lack of sleep can even mimic the aging process, making us look older before our time. And no woman likes to be told that she looks tired.

Sleep is the golden chain that ties health and our bodies together.

—Thomas Dekker

My friend Regina was so wrung out from the nonstop stress of building her public relations company that she decided she *had* to do something. She left the city, by herself, to rejuvenate at the Canyon Ranch spa. Instead of her normal strategy of exercising, she found herself drawn to the warmth of the fireside. Curled up in front of the crackling fire, lulled by its warmth, she fell into a deep, delicious sleep. During the day, she left her spot only to eat meals and attend a few cooking classes. It took her a full *six days* to catch up on her sleep, but she left feeling completely rested—a new person!

and so to bed

Getting enough rest helps us restore and honor our body. Because stress is the number one cause of insomnia, it's important to create soothing bedtime rituals. Follow these tips for a more sound sleep. You'll be glad you did.

- **Be predictable:** Go to bed around the same time every night, and try to get up at the same time each morning. Our bodies love routine.
- **Take a bath:** There's nothing like a warm bath to ease you into sleep.
- **Exercise early:** If you exercise, do it before dinner, not after. It can rev you up before bedtime.
- **Lower your "sleep debt":** If you've missed sleep or know you will have less time to sleep, such as a travel time change, get extra sleep in advance.
- **Nap or not:** Research has shown that strategic naps improve our performance and alertness.

- **Eat dinner early:** It's harder to sleep on a full tummy.

- **Deal with stress:** If troubles keep you awake, keep a journal by your bed to help you unburden your thoughts.

- **Save room for sleep:** Avoid paying bills, reading the paper, and other nonbedtime activities in your bedroom.

- **Turn off the television:** Watching TV before bed can seem relaxing, but it actually acts as a stimulant and disturbs our sleep. Curl up with a good book instead.

- **Go bland before bedtime:** To fall asleep more quickly, avoid caffeine, nicotine, and alcohol at least four hours before going to bed.

- **Grab a light snack:** It's hard to sleep if you're hungry. Try a light snack before bedtime if you're feeling hunger pangs. Some researchers think tryptophan, a chemical found in milk and turkey, naturally induces sleep. I find a banana or warm milk with honey helps me off to la-la land.

- **Get dark:** People usually sleep best in a cool, dark environment. (I swear by a soft eye mask that my mom specially made for me.) If necessary, invest in heavy drapes to keep out the early rays or the city's lights.

midlife maintenance

The most important part of honoring your body is knowing that you must be kind to it. Without taking care of your body, without strengthening it, without doing what you need to do to keep your body healthy, *you will not have the full life you want for yourself.* Your wants for yourself, your wants for others, your goals and aspirations, even the magic you want to share with the world—none of it can be fully realized without a strong, healthy body. Use your wisdom to fully grasp this truth.

You have a responsibility to keep your body healthy and strong. Be informed and inquisitive. Be proactive. Know what you need to do to maintain good health. And do it. Your body has a tremendous capacity to repair itself, but you can't expect the same resiliency at forty as you could at twenty. You must be aware of the challenges to your well-being, and you must learn how to fight back. It's important to have regular medical checkups throughout your life. Once you turn forty you should consider them mandatory maintenance. Many diseases and conditions can be treated successfully if discovered early enough, so it's up to you to respect yourself and assume responsibility for your own good health. Don't let a simple test or checkup come between you and your health. Don't let a simple test or checkup come between you and your future. Your loved ones will thank you for it.

cancer: Our risk increases as we get older. Fight back by:

- reducing fat
- eating whole foods high in antioxidants
- stopping smoking
- staying active
- drinking alcohol in moderation

diabetes: We're at risk if we're overweight and fifty. Fight back by:

- eating fewer processed foods
- eating more fiber-rich whole foods
- eating less fat
- staying active

heart disease: Near menopause we lose estrogen, increasing our risk of heart disease. Fight back by:

- reducing fat
- increasing fiber-rich fruits and vegetables
- eating more soy
- eating whole foods high in antioxidants
- stopping smoking
- staying active
- drinking alcohol in moderation

osteoporosis: Bone density decreases with age. Fight back by:

- increasing calcium—found in salmon, fortified cereals, and juices
- reducing caffeine from soft drinks, coffee, and tea
- engaging in weight-bearing exercises
- taking a calcium supplement with vitamin D (vitamin D aids in absorption)

Take care of yourself. Don't take your beautiful body for granted. Honor your body and give it the respect and recognition it deserves. Throw away the fad diets, the junk eating, and the couch potato lifestyle once and for all. Put yourself in motion and just begin. Take a walk and breathe the fresh air. Eat some veggies. Join a gym. Make an appointment for that physical you've been putting off. Mark "self-breast exam" on your calendar every month—and do it! Let's all of us get up off our tushies and proclaim, "I am going to do this *for myself.* And I'm going to do it, *today!*"

MIDLIFE MAINTENANCE

THE EXAM	HOW OFTEN
Blood Pressure Check	Once a year during a routine physical.
Bone Density Test	Once at the age of forty. If there are known risk factors, such as going through menopause without estrogen, a history of athletics, or if osteoporosis has been confirmed, speak with your physician concerning his or her recommendation for follow-up bone density exams.
Breast Exam	Once a month in the privacy of your home and once a year in your physician's office after the age of forty.
Total Cholesterol Check	Once every five years under the age of forty. From the age of forty, once a year.
Colon Exam	Every five years after the age of fifty.
Complete Physical	Once a year.
Dental Checkup	Once a year for a routine cleaning and every six months for a follow-up visit.
Eye Exam	Once every two years after the age of forty.
Mammogram	Once every two years beginning at the age of forty. Once every year after the age of fifty, especially if there is a history of breast cancer in your family.
Pap Test	Once every year, until you've had two normal tests one year apart, then once every two years. Or, once a year if there are known risk factors, such as a family history of cervical cancer, or a previous abnormal test.
Skin Exam	Once a year after the age of forty.

IF ANY SERIOUS HEALTH CONDITIONS RUN IN YOUR FAMILY, YOU WANT TO BE MORE VIGILANT WITH YOUR MEDICAL CARE.

Principle Four:
Discover Your Wisdom

**Draw on your experience
and know that you are wise**

By the time we reach midlife we have accumulated many experiences. We have felt joy and gladness. We've been sad. Sometimes we've been distressed. We have laughed and loved, and may even have lost ourselves in love. We have set out to build careers or raise families, sometimes all on our own. We've been moved by victories and touched by simple moments. We've felt overwhelming grief at the loss of loved ones, have endured humiliating defeats . . . and yet, amazingly, we have managed to build up our lives again. We have lived. We are alive!

The advantage is ours. We've had time to know what works and what doesn't and we need to realize that now we're sitting on an amazing bank of wisdom, a library of firsthand knowledge. Let's treasure it. Embrace it. Make the most of our hard-earned wisdom. Instead of thinking that we have lost worth by aging, that we are no longer young or viable, let's actively honor and appreciate the wisdom that age has brought us. Let's recognize that experience has made us better—and a whole lot wiser.

Growing up is an accomplishment. And it can take such a long time. So instead of thinking that we are "past it" or "over-the-hill," instead of reciting all those *shoulda, coulda, woulda* thoughts that hold us back, why not enjoy the freedom our experience has brought us? Why not take that know-how to help us live true? There isn't a better time.

Our teens and twenties were a period of testing and slowly establishing ourselves, a time to make our mark on the world and perhaps break away from what we felt was authority or restriction. Action was more important than contemplation. We were too busy to take inventory. And of course we couldn't see our patterns and tendencies then because we were in the process of creating them.

Admit that you are wise.

Acknowledge that your wisdom means freedom.

Above all, accept your wisdom.

Our thirties may have been spent raising families or developing careers, and sometimes, struggling to manage both. But for many of us, as we hit our mid to late thirties, after having tasted a bit of life, we reached a plateau, an in-between stage when we began to question what our lives were really about. We might also have been surprised to find that we still didn't quite feel grown up. We thought that, sometime, somewhere, someone was going to confer the status of grown-up upon us. Someday we would become that complete person who _____. (We can all fill in the blank about what it is we thought would make us complete and grown up.) We waited for that "official" confirmation. We waited through graduation, marriage, career success, motherhood, and we believed that one day we would finally be adults. Just not today.

Now, as we see forty and fifty staring back at us we may panic, thinking that we have somehow gone beyond that point of arrival. "Oh no," we fret. "Now I am my parents. Now I am old." And we ask, "Where did all the time go?" For many of us this mid-moment creates a sense of urgency, an insistent awareness that time is more important now than it ever was. And we don't want to waste it. When we were younger we felt that time was endless, that life would go on forever, and we were invincible. That's not true anymore. We know better now. We may feel as if we are thirty inside (we may believe that *forty is the new thirty*) but the calendar is telling us something else.

How can we make sense of this process of aging? How can we enter midlife with dignity when we don't have a clear idea of what the journey can look like, or what kind of person we can be at each age and stage? It's difficult, especially when everywhere we turn the media celebrates youth and tends to ignore a huge chunk of the population—us. It's enough to send us running backward in time to the security of the familiar years past.

I think we fear the unknown the most. That's natural. The years ahead haven't been modeled out for us yet, and we don't know what's in store. And while we may not know where we are going, we do know where we have been. Sometimes it can seem more reassuring to go back, to return to what we knew rather than face a future that is unknown. Maybe that's why some of us try to hold on to specific moments in our life when we felt we were at our best, our strongest. But we keep ourselves prisoners of the past when we do that.

Let's face it: growing older can bring losses. And losses can bring fear. But we mustn't let that fear pull us off course or make less of our natural evolution. We must learn to embrace each age if we are to live a life that's true. We must use our wisdom to appreciate the value of every age, and to find the courage to move forward into the unknown. Our life is an arc with a beginning, a middle, and an end. And we need to regard it—every moment—as something precious and complete. Think about it. How can any one part of life be less important than another? It is all our life, every moment good or bad. Every day is a gift. We must use our wisdom to claim every part of living and discover what is great about the age we are today. That's what is

> *That it will never come again is what makes life so sweet.*
> —EMILY DICKINSON

so wonderful about the Principles of Ageless Living—they provide us with the tools that we can use daily to support us at every age.

Uncover your wisdom. See where the truth lies and follow it. What was important to us at thirty cannot sustain us at forty or fifty. Know that. Move with it. Evolve with time and see how powerful and exciting this evolution can be. Let's look at our lives in the right light. Let's look at our lives as a whole and develop an understanding of the entire arc of life. Our journey brings gifts at each stage. There are treasures for us to discover at every age, opportunities that can be found now that aren't available to us at any other time in our life. It is important for us to know that all of life can be good and that possibilities await us at every turn. It is up to each one of us to find these treasures, seize these opportunities, and discover the value in the age we are right now.

Knowledge has a beginning but no end.

—GEETA S. IYENGAR

Wisdom is one of our treasures, and discovering that wisdom helps us to understand the benefits that come with age. We have more confidence now, more daring. We have more patience and compassion, and a better perspective on life too. And let's not forget that after all we've been through we have much more humor. By developing our wisdom, we can discover the newfound power those benefits bring. We have earned a deeper understanding of life, so let's use it to make better decisions, for ourselves and for those around us.

oh pioneer

We've all drawn inspiration from the daring discoverers and wise women who have expanded our understanding of the world. It probably started in grade school when we took out our scissors and scrapbook to paste stories of the women whose achievements helped shape our lives. Some of us may have been impressed by the intrepid Jane Goodall. Others will have been inspired by the personal integrity and athletic achievement of Wilma Rudolph, or the visionary wisdom of Barbara Jordan, who fought for an "America as good as its promise." There will be those of us who were drawn to the compassionate intelligence of Dian Fossey, to the wisdom and insight of Eleanor Roosevelt, or the audacity of Gloria Steinem. And likely there were many who looked to their stalwart mothers, their courageous sisters, and their spirited aunts.

That's wonderful. We all need people to look up to, and when we're young it's easy to draw on the wisdom of others. But whom do we look up to now that we have lived close to half our life? We can, of course, scrutinize those who came before us; there are so many wonderful people to learn from.

But think about it. Their lives were so very different from ours. Their experiences were different and so were their expectations. It's one thing to admire the accomplishments of the intrepid explorers, and to recognize the many firsts that have been achieved by the fascinating women who came before, but what about us? What about the goals that we want to accomplish during this, the second half of our lives? As midlife women whom do *we* look up to? Who can help us to be as good as *our* promise? The answer is closer that you think. . . .

Your future depends on many things, but mostly on you.
—FRANK TYGER

As midlife women we are living in an exciting time. We have the maturity and experiences to be our true selves, and now *we* have the opportunity to be the pioneers. No longer are we becoming, *it is time for us to be.* And as women of midlife at the beginning of the twenty-first century, each and every one of us has the opportunity to demand a new definition of the aging process, to change the face of midlife, and to determine the course of the rest of our lives. Instead of agreeing with the cultural message that life for us now has dwindling prospects, let's look at the possibilities, at the excitement that this phase of our life can bring. Let's be courageous and lead the way, become our own role models, and use our wisdom to create our accomplishments. The scrapbook belongs to us now, and it is up to

THE 5 PRINCIPLES OF AGELESS LIVING

us to fill it with stories of our own daring and wisdom. We must never forget that we have it in our power to make life continually exciting and enriching.

We really are explorers. We are creating new, positive ways of living today, and we are changing the face of aging, determining and creating our own lives for ourselves. We are reexamining how we want to spend our postworking years. We are asking our doctors for smoother transitions through menopause, and working to become—and stay—more physically fit longer. We are looking for more depth in our lives for the vital years ahead of us. We are becoming more audacious, less willing to accept what others tell us life should be. Midlife is giving us a much welcomed "who cares?" attitude. And that attitude, combined with our wisdom, is making this the time for us to dare, to go farther than we thought we could. We have less fear of failing now than we did when we were younger. Ask yourself, "Do I want to go through life regretting not having done things I clearly wanted to do?"

We have opportunities open to us as we get older that just would not have appealed to us in our younger years. We may be told over and over through the media that life offers us so much more when we are young, that opportunity dwindles as we enter into our later years, but I happen to believe the opposite! When we are young we start out with a lot of energy to launch ourselves into the world. And that's great.

But only with time can we develop a full, mature appreciation of life and be able to use that seasoned viewpoint to our advantage.

Our opportunities expand with age. When we draw from the rich base of our experiences we find that, with time, we have more of everything: more knowledge, more skills, more compassion. We have more humor and understanding.

If not now, when?
If not me, who?

We have perspective. At midlife, we have the wisdom to appreciate ourselves. We also have the wisdom to appreciate the full range of life's experiences. As I entered my forties I gained a sense of gratitude for the small things in life: unexpected kindnesses from a friend or a stranger, the warm spring sun on my face, the tang of the sea, the joy that I was alive. I took these things for granted when I was younger. I didn't have the wisdom to understand the immensity of the gifts I received each day. Now I realize that gratitude is an essential part of wisdom. And now that I have the wisdom to be grateful for what I have, I find I have the courage to go forward and create what I need.

holding patterns

Discovering our wisdom begins with living in a conscious way, noticing how we behave, how we treat others, how our actions resonate in the larger world. Living consciously is living with the intention to be our highest, each day. It is a lifelong practice, not an occasional impulse. When we live consciously we respond with awareness instead of just reacting to people and situations. It's important to look at life this way. So often we think that things *just happen*. Not so. When we are conscious of our actions, motives, and patterns we can understand ourselves better, as well as those around us.

Only when we recognize our patterns and understand our motives can we take more positive action in our lives. I've noticed again

The greater the challenge, the greater the treasure.

and again that when I'm not conscious, when I don't notice my habits and patterns, when I'm not clear about what I'm creating in my life by my thoughts and actions, I often end up with the opposite of what I want. That's when I wonder, "Why isn't my life turning out the way I wanted?"

I would say to anyone who complains that life keeps handing her the short end of the stick, "You get it until you *get it*." When we are called upon to evolve, as our challenges compel us to do, we must rise to the occasion. Our challenges are a gift for our growth, our evolution. That is why they come to us. The point is for us to find the gift hidden inside the challenge, to discover the treasure in each problem. And my experience in the gift is *always* there.

Midlife is the time to gather our gifts, to reclaim the parts of ourself that are stuck in the past. We need to let go of those trapped patterns below our awareness, and release them so that all our energies can flow in the same direction. We need to use our insight to become aware, our courage to be able to see, and our wisdom to make choices that support our highest self.

At midlife, we want more value in our life; we want to be our true self. Now, more than at any other time, we have the maturity and the courage to stop blaming circumstances and others for not having the kind of life we think we should have. It is up to us now. Using the lessons we've learned over time, we can pick up the reins of our life and bring it under our control. But if we are reluctant to learn the lessons that are there for us, if we allow our patterns to prevent our growth, the same difficult, challenging situations are likely to occur over and over again. The characters may change, the scenery may look different, but the circumstances stay the same—a sure sign of our own resistance.

When we don't notice our patterns we get in our own way. And how can we possibly move forward in life if we are bound by behavior we aren't even aware of?

For example, when we are criticized, we may get defensive instead of trying to hear the truth of what is being said. When this happens, an automatic cause and effect response kicks in, and over time, becomes a pattern we repeat mindlessly, without our awareness. The next thing we know, we have become a prisoner of this pattern, set off by a sort of knee-jerk reaction. In that moment we react, we are unconscious, and part of our life is unavailable to us. That time becomes lost time and we close ourselves off to the truth. But when we take the courage to look squarely at our patterns, when we unlock a negative habit or an automatic way of thinking, we are freed. Consider it: We can be set free just by becoming aware of our unconscious thoughts and involuntary actions. By getting to the root of those involuntary behaviors that have dictated our conduct for years, we can finally be free to find out what we are capable of on every level. How exhilarating!

Our patterns help reveal to us what we have chosen. They also tell us which parts of ourselves need recognition and a voice. Our inner voice needs to be heard. If we do not heed that voice, eventually we become depressed and risk internalizing disease. That is why it is so imperative to recognize our patterns now. We cannot live our true life by living out a suppressed personality. We cannot live our true life by avoiding intimacy. We cannot live our true life by staying stuck in oppressive situations, or by being afraid to dare to break out. Our patterns hold statements that dictate our unconscious behavior. They force us to react, without our awareness, in ways that may be completely untrue to us, and this can cause us tremendous suffering.

A few years ago I was working with a friend of mine on an assignment in a different city. The job was demanding and the deadline was tight, but Patty and I both found the work rewarding. We were very happy. One day, however, while Patty was focused on a particularly intense part of the project, she received an unexpected phone call from home. It was her sister. Acting as spokesperson for the rest of the family, Patty's sister conveyed their perception that she was ignoring her responsibilities at home, that she was "choosing her work over family obligations." Patty hung up the phone in a panic. Shaking and near tears, she decided on the spot that she had to go home. She must go home! I helped her calm down and we pieced the story together. "Here we go again. Everyone wants something from me," she said. "I can't be everything. I can't give each of them what they want and I'm just not good enough. No matter what I do, I'm not a good enough daughter. I'm not a good enough sister. I'm not a good enough girlfriend or employee." I urged Patty to take a few deep breaths, and then we talked about the concept of pat-

> *Inside yourself or outside, you never have to change what you see, only the way you see it.*
> —THADDEUS GOLAS

terns. Together we started to figure it out. Patty was the golden girl at home, the person everyone looked to for help. She liked this role, but at the same time felt constrained by it, and resented the fact that she could never do it all, no matter how hard she tried. And she tried *very* hard. Perhaps too hard. The fact was that somewhere, deep down, Patty believed that she had to be all things to all people, that it was her responsibility to save everyone. Hence her hot-button reaction.

Just taking a deep breath and a step back gave Patty the space to gather herself together. Thinking about the phone call and her reaction to it, she had the insight to realize that the conversation with her sister had put into play an old tape that she had been listening to for years, a tape she wasn't even aware she owned. But by taking the time to recognize the pattern, Patty could look at things more objectively and even see how she was participating in her own self-defeating behavior. She could take positive action by dealing with the situation at hand rather than the years of situations that had preceded it. Patty now has the insight and some tools to help dismantle her pattern, and the next time this situation comes up for her she will be able to respond more thoughtfully instead of mindlessly reacting when the panic button goes off.

It takes tremendous bravery to change, to go inside and realize you may be mistaken. It takes great courage to say, "You

know what, I was wrong," even to ourselves. It can be destabi-
lizing to admit that we might not be right. And frightening.
But when we do find the courage to acknowledge our mistakes
and take responsibility for a situation, we will be rewarded with
many gifts: a feeling of generosity, real power, and a rich and
honest humility. We feel our vastness when we are most humble. Our heart opens and we start connecting with our own

This is _your_ life. Everything you intend can be made manifest.

greatness. And only through wisdom and humility
can our greatness emerge. When we realize we're
capable of being wrong and take responsibility for
our actions we experience two waves of feeling:
humility in the first wave, and benevolence in the
second. And then we give room to greatness in our heart.

Midlife gives us the opportunity to look back on our
life and put things into perspective. We can realize where our
strengths lie and where we need to pay more attention. Now
is the time to forgive others, as well as ourselves, to look at
things in a larger context so that we may heal. Once that healing takes place, we can move forward. That said, it's important to recognize that _forgiveness, closure,_ and _moving forward_
can be buzzwords that may mask or trivialize what is actually
a complex, personal journey. It takes time for issues to develop
and it takes time to resolve them too. So don't rush forward.

Recognize that patience is sometimes a very important part of wisdom. Understand that healing is a process that unfolds over time—sometimes a long time.

writing your life

Journaling is one of the best ways I know to tap into wisdom. The simple act of writing down what we think and feel invites us to pause and be conscious of what it is we *are* thinking and feeling. Our lives are busy, and so often we act first and think later. It's only when we take the time to ponder something—"Why did this happen? Why did I say that?"—that our insights come. Journaling can give us that time. It can help us to discover how we feel, and it can also reveal and organize our thinking. What better way to truly get in touch with our wisdom?

Some women tell me they shy away from journaling because they aren't good at writing. I want to ask, "Who is grading us?" The point isn't to test our creative writing skills, but to explore what is on our mind and in our heart. Start journaling any way you can. But do start. Choose a lovely notebook and write in your journal by hand, type it on your computer, or speak into a tape. Or do all of the above. I love writing in a real journal, just like the diaries we kept as girls,

One way to get started journaling is to write down what comes to mind as you contemplate these thoughts:

- *What have I always wanted to do but never tried?*

- *What gives me joy? What gives me peace?*

- *What am I grateful for? Who am I grateful to?*

- *Who have my greatest teachers been?*

- *What are my fears and how can I conquer them?*

- *What would I like to change about my life?*

- *If I knew I wouldn't fail, what would I attempt to do?*

our secret book we poured our heart and soul into—but you should do whatever works best for you.

You can start your journal by making lists of what you really love to do and aren't in touch with, as my friend Mary Lou did. She said at first she was afraid to make a list. She had to step back a bit and really listen to know what she would even put on her list. But she said, "We *all* know that list, even if we are not in touch with it. Even children know that list." Remember, it was by making a list of what truly made her happy that helped Mary Lou access her wisdom and change her life completely.

A journal really can become a tool to create a better life. There is a group of women in Washington, D.C., called Suited for Change that helps women transition into the workforce from welfare and women's shelters. Survivors of some of life's toughest challenges, these women were encouraged by their workshop leaders to write journals as part of a development program. Working only with school-type spiral notebooks, markers, magazines, scissors, and glue, the women created their personal journals, decorating them with pictures and words that said more about their inner selves than their outward circumstances. (*O: The Oprah Magazine* was in special demand that day!) Today, more than a year later, these women are still keeping their journals—and still growing.

Journaling is breathing space on paper.

Once you're comfortable with journaling and the writing process you can think about going deeper and delving into some of the holding patterns we talked about earlier. Look back over your life and write down a recurring pattern you've noticed that you feel is holding you back and use the journaling process to bolster your efforts. You may, for example, have stayed in relationships that are not supportive, or noticed a recurring pattern of anger in your life. You may have a fear of standing up for yourself, or a tendency to constantly criticize those around you. Take your time to contemplate this tendency. Trust yourself. With some very honest soul-searching, you will recognize the pattern that holds you back. Remember that you are wise.

- Write down three ways that you can take positive action about this tendency. Read over your choices several times. Choose the one that seems the best. Close your eyes. Imagine yourself back in a situation where you felt that negative tendency. Think of the people involved and their reactions to you at the time. Try to remember how acting in this old way made you feel.

- Now imagine yourself acting in the new positive way. Try to visualize how the same people involved would respond to your new choice of behavior. Write down the scenario and see how it plays out.

- Draw the story out a little farther; follow the impact of this positive behavior and visualize how it makes you feel afterward. Notice how much more love you feel for yourself and for all the people involved.

- Take a moment to say a short prayer, asking for the support to put into action your new positive intentions.

- Make notes of the tendency you are working on and the ways you want to handle it. (Post-its are great for this.) Display them in your home and office—even in the car. Just be sure to post them where they will always be visible.

- Look for opportunities during the day to practice the intentions you have recorded in your journal. You might practice patience if you are standing in line at Starbucks (there are *always* lines).

- Before you go to sleep, write in your journal the times you succeeded in behaving in new ways. Note why you were able to remember to put them into action, and how you felt afterward. Also, note the moments you feel you missed an opportunity to put them into practice and why.

- Review your day in your mind. Give thanks for being able to succeed at making the change. If you found you couldn't make the change, don't worry. Be kind to

POST YOUR POSITIVE INTENTIONS

Breathe!

It will work out.

Sit up straight.

You don't have to do it all.

Take a break.

You are good.

See blessedness in every event.

Follow the joy!

yourself. This is a process and you will eventually succeed. Renew your intention to continue tomorrow. Be conscious, watchful, in the present, so that you can continue to replace your negative tendencies with positive ones.

- Once you feel you have successfully broken one bad habit you can start working on a second one. Look over your life once again for another pattern that may be holding you back, and repeat the previous process until you feel you have again succeeded.

As wise women, regular contemplation through journaling keeps us in tune with what might be limiting us, but more importantly, with what can free us. Journaling helps to clarify what we need to pay attention to, and it reminds us that we *can* take action to make our own lives better. A few things to bear in mind:

- *Be gentle with yourself.* Don't be self-critical or harsh. *No judgments.* Discovering our wisdom is intended to help us be better friends with ourselves and others, better partners, and better people.

- *Forgive yourself for any slipups.* Our tendencies took a lifetime to develop, so it will take a continued, gentle vigilance to make a difference.

- *Give yourself time.* Discovering our own wisdom is a constant process of being present and aware. If we are honest with ourselves, we will be able to replace our negative tendencies with positive ones!

One more thing. Don't think that journaling is just about delving into the past. It can also help us to explore the future. A journal can help you become clear about what you truly want in your life *and* help you to create it. My friend Cheryl Richardson is a successful "life coach" who has written several very helpful books about the practical ways women can realize the life they want. Cheryl believes that a journal is essential for personal development and a great tool to connect to inner wisdom. She also knows that writing in her own journal changed her life. Several years ago when Cheryl was single and wanted to find a special person to share her life, she decided to create a profile of her ideal partner in the pages of her journal. Shortly after, she had a dream of a man standing on a platform high above her, presenting something to her. She wrote it all down in her journal. Nine months later Cheryl met a very nice man who seemed very familiar to her, but she couldn't quite place him. It was not until he showed her the house that he was constructing and happened to walk out onto the floor above—a platform—to present the upstairs of his home that it finally hit her. He was the man she had dreamt of! Cheryl raced home and grabbed her journal. The event she had just experienced was the scene she had written, and she had described it exactly. The man— Michael—looked exactly as she had depicted him in her journal nine months before. Think there's a happy ending to this story? You're right. Cheryl and Michael got married!

body of knowledge

So often when we use the word "wisdom" we think of things that are intellectual, of matters of the mind rather than matters of the heart or soul. But it's important to recognize that as wise women we are a composite of all the experiences we've accumulated: the emotional, the spiritual, the intellectual—and the physical. So why not take the time to appreciate and explore the satisfying physical pleasures of our wisdom? We've certainly earned them.

Sex means different things to different people, so it can be challenging to discuss. Nevertheless, sex *is* part of living a full and true life, so it can't be ignored. Sex, intimacy, and our close relationships are all tied to the many experiences that we've had. It's important to realize that. It's equally important to realize that these experiences have made us stronger and wiser, better able to make the right choices. We need to have the wisdom to recognize that at this time in our lives we do have a lot of choices. We've found out the hard way what works and what doesn't, and we need to use the wisdom of our experiences to open ourselves up to what we want and what we need. And do something about it.

Sex at midlife can be wonderful. Of course it's different for everyone, just as it was when we were younger, but there is no reason that we can't have a vital and healthy sexual life at every stage—at forty, fifty, sixty, and beyond.

> Our body has a wisdom all its own.

Sex is communication. It's an important part of a loving connection with another person, and when it's great—which it can be!—it's also a wonderful way to communicate emotionally and spiritually. But we can only communicate when we make ourselves available, and sometimes at midlife we get caught in a rut and forget just how glorious and fun sex can be. We may feel too busy to be up for it at the end of the day. We may not think we look good enough, and that can make us feel vulnerable and unattractive. We may be dissatisfied with our relationship. We may feel that things have become monotonous and sex itself just a routine, or perhaps if we've been single for a while we may doubt the prospect of a romantic relationship. We may even think that "it's over" for us. But it doesn't have to be that way.

It's important to stay open to the possibilities that surround us. It's important that women over forty know that it's not over for them. I hear this all the time. "Oh, it's too late for me." "I'll never find anyone at my age." "All the good ones are taken." This is simply not true, so don't make it true by believing in it. Take away the power of those stale old statements. Part of being wise is believing in your worth and in the value of what you have to offer. Yes, there are men who only want to be with younger women (sometimes much younger women). There

Let's face it. We've been living in our bodies for a while. We know who we are and what we want. We're less self-conscious, and at midlife most of us are more daring. At this stage of our lives we feel confident to voice our needs and desires, more entitled to go after what we want. This is a good time.

are men, probably a lot of them, who, for whatever reason, think they need a second chance with someone younger than they are—someone younger than you. Don't let their problem become your problem. Know that there are many men (good men, honest men) who are looking for the same thing you are: a close and committed relationship with a loving partner. Open yourself up to the possibility.

It can be difficult to be alone when you want to have a partner, someone special in your life whom you can call anytime and just simply say, "Hi, it's me." If you've been in a long-term relationship and it's broken up—the statistics on this can be pretty frightening—being on your own again can be terrifying. But know that being without a partner doesn't have to mean the same thing as being alone. Know that the bed can be half full rather than half empty. Use this "by yourself" period to develop other things in your life. Commit this time to taking care of yourself, to working on your body and your mind. Develop a business, learn to play the piano, or sleep till noon on Sundays. Whatever you want.

> *Things come suitable to their time.*
> —Enid Bagnold

A romantic relationship needs time, and if you're not in a relationship right now enjoy that time to cultivate a better relationship with yourself and those around you. This is when you really need to connect with friends and family and community. Rely on your friends. Turn to your family. And tap into the strength you know you have. As scary as this time may be, use it to discover other parts of yourself that you might not have had access to before. Believe in yourself and in your own power to get what you want and what you need. And know that sometimes they aren't the same thing. Be patient and understand that this might be the time for you to be on your own. No one knows what tomorrow will bring. But if we're doing all the right things, if we're engaging in life and being true to who we are, then our wisdom and our courage will come through in trusting that we will have what we need.

Midlife is the time when we can finally own our desires. Chances are, when we first experienced sex we were very keen on pleasing our partner, keen to do the "right thing." Now that we've lived a little we're probably freer with our own needs, more willing to take ourselves into consideration. It can be difficult for women to put themselves first, though, to say "This is what I want, this is what I need." Nevertheless, acknowledging our needs is vital to discovering our wisdom, and expressing it too. It's part of taking responsibility for who we are. We can't live a true life unless we stand up and admit to ourselves what we truly need. But that can be scary. Because once we've admitted our needs to ourself, it's up to us to communicate those needs to the people we are close to. That doesn't mean that we should voice every whim or indulge every fancy; it simply means acknowledging what we need to make ourselves happy.

A great relationship is built by satisfying our own

Desire, ask, believe, receive.

—STELLA TERRILL MANN

needs as well as those of our partner. Only then can we use our physical selves to satisfy the intimate or spiritual part of sex, the part that can be transforming. Unfortunately, as women the conditioning is strong for us to acquiesce. Often we feel that after giving so much to everybody, somebody somewhere is going to notice and eventually it will become "our turn." We give and give and give in so many aspects of our life that we find it difficult to let go of our responsibilities and become deliciously self-interested. Nevertheless, whether we are starting a new relationship or revitalizing an old one, it's important that both partners have their needs met. Of course there's always an area of compromise—let's be real—but if things are out of balance then it's just not going to work. Sex can be a proving ground for a relationship. When problems rumble below the surface we may not feel able to meet them head-on, but often they manifest themselves sexually, either as a lack of desire or a pulling away. When we don't feel heard, or don't dare to voice our needs, we tend to shut down. We may still function well enough, but we can become isolated, possibly withdrawn. We may even become depressed. We hold back on intimacy and we hold back on life. But when we feel confident within ourselves and steady with our partners, when we feel that the relationship is safe and reciprocal, then we also feel able to say what it is that we need. I mean *really* need. When we accept the wisdom that is born of experience, it gives us the courage to dare. It gives us the freedom to say what we want, and if sometimes it's right to say "No. Not this . . ." so be it. That's what is so great about this time of life. It's our time. This is when it all comes together, when desire and wisdom meet. And boy, can it be great!

the power of passion

Life without passion can make us feel fed up and listless. And yet we often defer our passions—we haven't got the time, we have too many responsibilities, we're too old to start something new. But ask yourself: Do you really want to live a life without passion? We all need to find what it is that excites us, what it is that puts the zing in our life and makes our heart go *pitta-pat.* That which is closest to our heart inspires and renews us, giving us more energy to direct toward other parts of our life. It is never too late to learn something new, something we may feel we haven't had the time or resources to follow. When we pursue what we enjoy, we ignite passion in our lives, awakening the possibilities in our daily routine and adding excitement to our lives. Finding a new passion opens up our world and adds to our bank of wisdom. It makes us come alive.

Instead of simply riding the roller coaster of life, the ups and downs that are a part of our day, we need to create more room in our life for passionate pursuits, for those moments that can help us get lost in what we really love. It's time to remember that by losing ourselves, we often *find* ourselves.

When we find something new—or old—that we have passion for, and we follow that impulse, we simply renew our excitement, giving ourselves new energy to leap back into our lives.

Passion gives us energy that we can invest in our relationships. When we are happy, when we are doing what we love, then others benefit as well. It may sound selfish on the surface, but in fact, pursuing our own happiness has a direct impact on everyone around us, in all forms; love, friend-ship, even work, are all directly related to our personal sense of happiness and well-being. Even a small improvement in our own sense of well-being can work wonders on our ability and willing-ness to give to those around us.

Passion and wisdom go hand in hand. Our passion leads us toward wisdom, in turn making us wiser.

How can we discover our passions? We can start by revisiting the things we were enthusiastic about as a child. Midlife is a wonderful time to pick up the threads in our life that we may have let go: painting, drawing, arts and crafts, playing an instrument, reading, poetry, games—all the things we used to love but felt we never had time for. Now we can begin to make the time.

Pursuing a subject that interests us or trying something we've never done before may also blossom into a passion. On a whim, my friend Pam signed up for a university course on medicine for laymen that she saw listed in the newspaper. An author used to descriptive language and the magic of writing, she was surprised to find that she loved the challenge of thinking in a different way—scientifically. Suddenly, she found a new passion in science. Another woman I know (let's call her Jane) decided she needed to make a bold move when her husband's job relocated them from Washington, D.C., to Connecticut and she had to leave her own job—at the CIA! Exploring her passion for reading romance novels, she attended a Romance Writers Convention just for the fun of it. That's how she discovered her passion for *writing* romance novels. She's had two books published so far. Who knew?

What is passion? It is surely the becoming of a person.

—JOHN BOORMAN

Your own passion may also ignite someone else's passion as well. While I was in New Mexico for a women's conference, my friend Deb took me with her to the local photo galleries. It reminded me of my own love for photography. Deb has always been interested in photographs and recently signed up for her third year at the New School in New York for evening classes to learn about collecting photography. Along

THE 5 PRINCIPLES OF AGELESS LIVING

with the other students, she will find herself in a photo studio one day, at an art dealer's another, or visiting a private collection. Photography has become a passionate hobby for her, as well as being both social and educational. Deb's passion has led her to build a wonderful collection, while extending her knowledge of the art through her classes and the Web. It's also a way she can share with her friends. I often get a call about the latest photo show we must see together. Through her own passion, Deb has also rekindled mine!

the value of effort

It takes courage to see what we create, the good and the bad. It takes a brave soul to search inside and come up with the truth, especially since some of our patterns and motives might not be so flattering. We might not like what we see. But with courage, discipline, and wisdom—with good old-fashioned effort—we can discover how some of our unconscious demeanors might hold a key to why we are struggling in some areas of our life. Noticing our behavior and really examining it is not for the faint of heart. But if we want to live a true and valuable life, if we really want to take control of our life, then we have to put forth the effort to tap into our wisdom and see what we are made of. Discovering our wisdom takes effort. But my experience has been that when we harness a devoted effort, we find grace enters our life. Consider it: When we work toward our own betterment, as well as the betterment of others, we actually attract grace. When we act free from expectations and personal interest, our wisdom comes to us in the form of insights; and when we have insight into our life we create an opening for growth. Just as in a cartoon, when a lightbulb comes on over the character's head and out of the blue he has a realization, we too have "lightbulb" moments, openings in our life when, suddenly, we see things differently in a more expanded light. This is how grace, or the "descent of grace," works.

Self-effort and grace are like the two wings of a bird.

—SWAMI MUKTANANDA

Some of us may regard grace as good fortune, as a kindness, or perhaps a blessing. I understand grace as God's compassion, which is a teaching of Eastern thought. It doesn't really matter what we call it, though; what matters is that we understand that we all have the capacity to experience grace as an "inner unfolding" of the possibilities within us. But don't think that this process of unfolding can happen all by itself: the role of our own effort is invaluable. Grace needs our help. Grace can come into our lives only when we prepare for its arrival. I like to think of this process as tilling a field, where our effort is the actual preparation of the ground, allowing it to receive the blessings that will come our way. The rain, the sun, and even the seeds come from somewhere else. It is a partnership—a partnership with God. We need to be aware of grace working in our life, even in the smallest way, and to find the means to express our gratitude for all we have. Feeling gratitude for the grace that comes into our life enhances all our experiences, allowing us to see joy in the smallest moments.

give it a try

Our wisdom has many points of entry, many paths to reach what lies inside. I have found that when I put forth the effort to do the things I've dreamed of, things that to me are new and untried, I discover wisdom I didn't even know I had. We all can access hidden parts of ourselves by delving into new experiences, especially in areas we may have been afraid of. These parts lie dormant just waiting for the opportunity to be revealed. By challenging ourselves, we develop the wisdom we *already* have. The more we explore our restrictions, the more we build our resources and the more confident we become to take life on.

You'll be surprised by how much more vitality is available to you now (especially if you're taking good care of yourself), and how much more energy you will release if you do follow your passion. Take the first steps to liberate yourself from the feeling that you are under-living your life. Tap into your wisdom. Challenge yourself to try what you have never before attempted and great energy will follow. Try it. Give yourself a chance to ignite a spark. Dare yourself to do something you may have been too frightened or self-conscious to attempt. It doesn't matter whether it's starting a business, pursuing a long-hidden dream, or just enrolling in an evening class. What matters is that you try.

My mother is talented in so many areas, but growing up she didn't have a lot of faith in her abilities. In her fifties, with her family grown, she realized that raising four children and running a household had fostered her gift for management and organization. She started managing a small medical office and was so successful at it that today she runs all the office work and billing for fifty-three doctors. And they can't get along without her. She works five days a week, nine to five, and doesn't seem to be slowing down. She has a newfound sense of pride and confidence in herself and says the work keeps her young. By the way, did I mention that my mom, Terry, is now almost eighty?

We all need to find ways to recharge and keep ourselves young, to continue to learn and grow. There are so many possibilities,

> **We are a bundle of restrictions seeded on greatness.**

so much to discover. You may have thought your secret wish to learn painting, make pottery, or design jewelry was silly, and pushed it back to the recesses of your mind. Get rid of the word *silly*, and silence the voice that tells you that you missed your chance. There is no such thing. And there is no better time to open up the possibilities of a long-dormant passion. If you have put off traveling, now is the time to explore and broaden your vision. If you have neglected a hobby or passion, now is the time to rekindle that interest. Who knows? You may even turn that pastime into a new business!

> *What you are is God's gift to you. What you do with what you are is your gift to God.*
> —GEORGE FOSTER

a class act

Midlife is a great time to go back to school and get a degree or pursue a dream we may have abandoned or deferred. Continuing our education, whether finishing a degree or just taking a class, invigorates more than our mind; it reawakens our connection to the world, adds to our bank of wisdom, and expands our horizons. When we discover new avenues of wisdom, we become worldly. And when we know more *of* the world, we are more *in* the world. In this way, we become wiser, and through our wisdom, connected to others. When we reconnect with subjects like world history, science, and religion, we become aware of our place in the larger world. Feeling uplifted by the genius that created great music, art, and literature, we are inspired to do great things in our own lives.

My friend Barbara went back to school to earn her art history degree when she was in her forties. She was the oldest person in the class. At first she felt awkward because of the age difference, but soon she became the one the younger students turned to for advice about life. Barbara got her degree. She accomplished something important for herself that gave her a renewed sense of energy and confidence. And along the way she found an unexpected joy in being able to give of herself to others.

I expect I shall be a student to the end of my days.

—ANTON CHEKHOV

My sister Darilyn is an extraordinary person, always giving. I admire her very much. While working at a crisis clinic, she was so moved by the many injustices women suffered that she decided to do something about it. Studying at night, she earned her law degree while raising two children and holding down a full-time job. The oldest in her class (she was in her fifties at the time), Dari had to confront her extreme shyness when standing up and speaking in front of people less than half her age. Today, Dari is helping women in need. She tapped into her wisdom to extraordinary results. Not only has she gained more confidence in herself and her abilities, she also took the initiative to go after something she was passionate about. But there's more. Daring to take on her own development and enhance her wisdom, Dari inspired her daughter Zephora to further her own growth. Just thirty and a mother of a toddler, Zephora had been thinking of getting her masters in international relations but was sitting on the fence. When Dari went ahead with her decision to get a law degree, Zephora thought, "If my mom can do it, I can do it too." So she put aside her hesitation and went back to school. Zephora says that even though she finds it exhausting to raise her active little boy full-time *and* study at night, it saves her life as a mother. "My brain is nourished and I feel inspired. Yes, it's hard, but the gains far outweigh the difficulties. It's such a departure from what I do during the day that it refreshes me as a parent. And I wouldn't have done it without my mom's example."

Formal learning is great for developing discipline and confidence, encouraging mental agility, and helping us put things in their proper perspective. We may even share our wisdom by mentoring younger students, as Barbara did, or inspiring others, as Darilyn did. Sharing is a big part of discovering our wisdom, so why not take things one step further and share a class with a friend? It can be a creative way to learn something new while spending time with someone you care about. My friend Regina and I recently took cooking classes at the Culinary Institute in New York. We spent five days with a small dedicated group, some of whose members had traveled from out of state. One young woman was learning to cook so that she could surprise her fiancé with a romantic dinner. Another couple wanted to gain knowledge so that they could cook together. During the week, we learned some of the basics of French cooking; how to julienne vegetables, whip up soufflés, prepare lamb the French way, fold an *omelette aux fines herbes,* and manage a mouthwatering chocolate mousse. After cooking each day we all sat around the kitchen table to taste what we had so proudly made. It was great fun. Not only did we meet wonderful people who shared our interest, but we acquired new skills that Regina and I both use. Our cooking experience excited and rejuvenated us so much that we sign up for new classes whenever we can. And I can now make a mean crème brûlée!

> *To be tested is good. The challenged life may be the best therapist.*
> —GAIL SHEEHY

■ ■ ■

At midlife, we often have the drive to enjoy wisdom for wisdom's sake. We can become empowered as we expand our understanding. We can find courses and degree programs by contacting community colleges or universities. Many schools have adult courses, at night or on weekends. Ask about special "back to school" programs, part-time degrees, and noncredit classes. You can even go to school on-line. It doesn't have to be complicated. I recently discovered Fathom, an on-line learning community that features professors from some of the top universities (see Resource Guide). You can take courses on anything from the Civil War to Buddhism. Some courses are free, others are modestly priced; they range from a single lecture to a semester-long course. Cooking schools, museums, institutes, and even some hospitals are all good places to find classes. If you want to learn public speaking with confidence, try Toastmasters. And if you just want to experiment with something new, try the many nonacademic courses that are offered at the Learning Annex. It's a great adult education resource that provides learning opportunities from amateur photography to massage to wine-tasting (see Resource Guide). One of my friends even learned how to read auras from a Learning Annex class!

Lessons and workshops are one route to our hidden talents. But we can also uncover talents without lessons: from books, magazines, videos, computer software, even kits. There are as many opportunities available to us as we have interests: writing workshops, sculpting classes, dance classes, jewelry design, and more to choose from at your community center. AARP offers an abundance of opportunities through its newest publication, *AARP: The Magazine,* all of which you can put to use to bring out *your* own hidden talent. And we all have one (or two!). So start humble and start local. Just be sure to start.

read

Sometimes the easiest way to learn is just by opening a book. I'm always enchanted with the idea that a good book can stimulate my thinking and open up a new world, right before my very eyes. We can all access our wisdom by reading books on any subject imaginable. I enjoy books on spirituality because I'm always interested in more profound ways to look at the world. I like Aristotle, Voltaire, and Shakespeare (not exactly light reading, but they can be a joy for the senses and a spark plug for the mind), and I also enjoy Anna Quindlen, Anita Shreve, Anne Morrow Lindbergh, and *any* great biographies. I like to suit my book to my mood—a heavy book when I'm in a somber mood, a light read for the beach, or perhaps a short story when I'm looking for a brief diversion. Our tastes change, so it's important to be open to our need for variety. From poetry to contemporary novels, from philosophy to the classics, each has something to offer—and something to ask. I'm always amazed at how relevant some of the older books are. They may have been written several hundred years ago; nevertheless their concerns seem timeless and relevant even today.

As wise women, we want to understand ourselves as best we can. Books enrich us, so that we can live more fully. I find that self-help books, which are available in just about every subject, guide us through many of our challenges and show us how to better understand ourselves. Throughout my life, I have turned to books over and over again to teach myself something new or to learn how other people have experienced their life and faced their challenges. I love the way that books can move me to tears or laughter, or just transport and entertain me. I adore books and always have. (I was my high school librarian just so that I could read as much as I wanted!)

If you'd like to connect with others and dive into a great book at the same time, join a book group. You'll be able to expand your horizons and meet like-minded people. Book groups are great because they often suggest titles you might not have heard of. Take a chance. Wander into a part of the bookstore you've never been in before. Try different kinds of books. I know that my horizons opened up by reading about World War II inspired by my dad who fought in the war. See if a new world opens up for you. Books hold the power to add to wisdom we already have. So, put down your TV remote and get thee to a library or bookstore!

learn a new language

It's never too late to learn a language. A friend's mother in her fifties decided to take French lessons when her daughter moved to Paris. Once she learned French, she was inspired to take French cooking classes. That led her to study French culture, and that led her to strengthen her connection with her daughter.

Learning a foreign language opens up worlds for us. When we are able to connect with people in their own language, we feel adventurous and playful. Language classes are also a wonderful way to meet new people. Go with a friend so you can practice on each other. Some ways to get started:

- *Teach yourself* courses on audio, videotape, and CD-ROM.
- Classes on the Internet, through museums, and the Y.

CHILD'S PLAY

Learning a language doesn't have to be all work and no play. To learn Italian, I started with books for two- and three-year-olds, and then progressed to age five, six, and seven. Children's books are colorful, an easy way to learn more quickly, and much more fun. *Adesso è possibile anche per te. Arrivederci. Buona fortuna!!*

- Language schools, such as Berlitz.
- Sing along with your favorite CD—Edith Piaf or Bocelli.
- High schools often have language teachers who can direct you to a tutor.
- Plan a trip to a place you've always wanted to go, then prepare by learning the language.

passport to wisdom

Getting a passport, even if you haven't scheduled a trip, might be just what you need to give you the wanderlust to travel. A passport can open up possibilities and become your doorway to freedom, as it did in my friend Michele's case. Michele didn't have a reason to travel out of the country.

Traveling abroad for her seemed exotic, something other peo- ple did. But recently, when she decided to join some friends on a trip they were taking, she realized she needed a pass- port. Not one for red tape, Michele was so pleasantly sur- prised when she found out how easy it was to get her own passport that she quickly got one for her husband and twelve- year-old son—"just in case." Getting a passport gave Michele a new sense of adventure, a liberating feeling that anything was possible. With her passport in hand she has visited Lon- don, Paris, and Florence. And last year she finally convinced her husband to join her in Europe—and he *loved* it. Something that seemed out of reach became real simply because Michele got a passport before she even knew where she was headed.

As a woman, my country is the whole world.

—VIRGINIA WOOLF

Travel can be our most direct route to adventure. When I was growing up I was sure of one thing: I wanted to see the world. Though I come from Canada, I feel an enor- mous connection with all the places I've spent time in: France (where I lived for ten years), the United States (where I've lived for more than fifteen years), Italy, Denmark, and India. Every chance I've had to see the world has only given me more insights and more gifts. Inside of me live all the sights, the people, the languages I've experienced. They are a tremendous resource to draw upon when I come home. I carry them with me, always.

We may see obstacles to travel—expense, time, language, fear, or not having travel companions. It may take effort on our part, but none of these issues have to hold us back. The rewards far outweigh the challenges. Besides the usual resources—travel agents, travel Web sites, the airlines—there are many other avenues to plan trips. Some museums, like New York's Metropolitan Museum of Art, organize fantastic trips led by scholars. Magazines such as *Yoga Journal* offer exciting trips to the Far East, combining yoga with history. Colleges and universities arrange trips—for both alumnae and nonalumnae—led by faculty members. Or connect with your church group for a travel adventure together, or any of your local groups that might have a secret desire to explore.

Go on a cruise. Go on a bus trip, even if it's just for a day. You can venture near, you can venture far. You can go alone, or with a friend. But travel! It opens up your world and gives you adventure.

discover a hidden talent

A friend of mine always wanted to learn horseback riding as a child but her parents couldn't afford it. At midlife, she realized with delight that *she* could. The financial security that came with maturity enabled her to make her childhood fantasy a reality. She began taking lessons at a local park stable and discovered the pleasure of finally doing something she'd always wanted to do. In addition to the personal gratification of fulfilling her childhood dream, riding allowed her to develop a deep connection with animals. The process of learning to communicate with and understand her horse brought her to a fuller understanding of herself. And by approaching this long-desired pastime with the wisdom of midlife, she gained a sense of peace and confidence.

Another friend, Kandy, had a secret wish: to sing. And at midlife, she decided to do something about it. Kandy found a voice teacher. She got herself a microphone and an amplifier, and for one year she practiced and practiced and practiced. Sometimes her friends would join her. We would all end up in her singing room, and with sheet music in hand, would take turns to indulge our own diva fantasies. Most of the time we would be on the floor howling with laughter over the "show."

Kandy made a commitment to herself, as well as a promise to her husband, to fulfill her wish of singing publicly. She finally got her chance. She would debut on a cruise ship in an impromptu little show put together by the staff and passengers on board. Thinking it was to be an intimate gathering around a piano, and encouraged by her husband, Kandy agreed to do it. But, when the evening came around, Kandy realized as she watched each performer go on before her, that the event was growing bigger and bigger. She just wanted to disappear. The other performers were professionals. She was the only amateur. The "little evening by the piano had become an extravaganza," she said, "with big stars and little me." Kandy wanted to get out of it but felt she had given her word. On top of it, her husband, sick with a high fever, had gotten out of bed to cheer her on. How could she *not* do it? The moment arrived to go on and Kandy was terrified, "shaking all over." She thought, "Thank God it is dark and I'm blind as a bat, so I don't have to see anyone." The orchestra began her song and Kandy froze. Listening to the first few bars of the music, she thought, "Wow! They sound great." She lost her focus and the band started without her. When she finally leaped into the

At midlife, we all have talent. We all have wisdom. When we discover one, we reveal the other.

song she found she was behind the music. The musicians kept on playing, hoping that she would catch up, but no matter how hard they tried, orchestra and singer couldn't get in sync. Thank goodness for the emcee. He stopped the music and addressed the audience: "This woman's got a great voice. Let's start over again." The audience roared its approval. Kandy, encouraged by the response, took a deep breath and started once more. This time, it was perfect. Timing, orchestra, melody, voice, and huge applause—*perfect.*

Afterward, Kandy admitted that the pain of flubbing hit her right in the stomach. "But I got through it and that was wonderful. People liked my voice," she said. "I did it. And I can do it again!"

Learning is movement from moment to moment.

—J. KRISHNAMURTI

Since then, Kandy has been singing regularly at her community center. She brings a lot of pleasure to those who hear her, and I'm happy to say that she's in step with herself and in time with the music. Kandy took a chance and uncovered a hidden talent. She created a whole lot of fun for herself—and for others—and has added another dimension to her wisdom.

■ ■ ■

I love the stories of courage and chutzpah that always seem to
unfold when women discover their hidden talents, whether
they are on a mission or just on a lark. As these stories tell us,
it takes just a little effort to gain so much. At midlife, we are
at the best time to fulfill our dreams and accomplish what we
have always wanted. We now have more confidence,
resources, common sense, and initiative than at any other
time in our lives. It's time for us to *shine*. Our talent—and our
wisdom—can take us anywhere.

Principle Five: Stay Connected

Reach out to family, friends, and community

Each of the five Ageless Living Principles is a call to act with awareness. We look our best when we consciously take care of our appearance. We nurture our spirit when we knowingly nourish the divine aspects of ourselves. We honor our body when we consciously care for it. We discover our wisdom when we tune in to the lessons of our experience. And when we purposefully and consciously come together with others, when we make the most of each moment and understand the power we have in us to put truth into action and engage with other people, then we stay connected.

the circle is unbroken

Feeling connected to others is a great source of joy. When we reach out to others, and they to us, we experience love in our life. Our links to family, friends, and community are vital for our sense of belonging and well-being. They create a safe haven. They offer us the opportunity to give of ourselves, and to be ourselves. When we lose this connection, we suffer. When we don't have warm, loving relationships, we feel disconnected and isolated from the world. We may even withdraw. Without supportive ties, we can begin to doubt ourselves, feeling negative about our place in the world and pessimistic about our possibilities. Feeling bad, we retreat. We make our world smaller. We begin to sever connections. Isolation then becomes the glue that keeps our hurts in place. By putting up barriers and separating ourselves from life around us, we linger within our negative experiences rather than moving beyond them. We replay them over and over, increasing their magnitude and consequently increasing our own loneliness and lack of connection. We may even convince ourselves that we are victims.

Loss of connection has an impact on our health and well-being and can ultimately make us feel old before our time. Conversely, staying connected can literally add *years* to our lives. In Okinawa, Japan, people live longer than anywhere else in the world. The average lifespan for women is eighty-four-plus years compared to an average of seventy-nine years for American women. Much has been made of the Okinawan's diet (they thrive on mainly fish, vegetables, rice, and soy), but researchers also cite the islanders' strong sense of community as one of the secrets to their longevity.

Okinawans embrace the idea of what they call *yuimaru*, from the Japanese word meaning "circle" or "connection." It refers to a sense of belonging and feeling important, being necessary to the larger community. Okinawans believe that *yuimaru* is vital to making people want to wake up in the morning and be productive. They believe that everyone is an essential link in the community and generational chain, so all the generations stay connected to each other, supporting and celebrating each other throughout their lives. The connections are real and meaningful. Neighbors are like family. Everyone comes together to do a service, whether it's to build a house or raise crops. Even building the family tomb is a community experience. For the Okinawans, *yuimaru* is more than a tradition, it's a way of life. The value and importance of nurturing and maintaining connections with everyone in the community is proven by the long, healthy lives they have as a result.

Call it a clan, call it a network, call it a tribe, call it a family. Whatever you call it, whoever you are, you need one.

—JANE HOWARD

By contrast, in the U.S., where we often don't share that sense of community, research shows that lack of connection causes depression and can even lead to physical debilitation. Adults who are dissatisfied with the amount of social support in their lives are more likely to suffer from depression than those with stronger social ties. In addition, as a 1996 study in *Psychology and Aging* showed, adults aged sixty-five and older who undergo some kind of physical impairment often feel a decrease in *perceived* social connection. Feeling disconnected can take its toll on our minds and emotions, as well as our bodies.

When we reach out and connect to those around us, we reverse this process. By being aware of the larger picture, one that includes all the people in our life, we put our personal moments in perspective. We recognize that we are part of a greater whole—and that recognition is empowering. We open up our capacity to love when we reach out to others. Instead of being filled with anger, fear, and anxiety, we are able to turn toward actions that fill us with compassion and grace, allowing us to renew our spirit and soar.

After the September 11 terrorist attack in New York, a city where isolation is the norm, I saw people making an immediate shift toward concern for one another. Everyone was reaching out to comfort strangers. Lines to donate blood stretched around the block, and crowds of people willing to volunteer their time were so large that many had to be turned away. The city rallied so quickly that it was hard to handle the influx of generous giving. Everyone just wanted to help and contribute in any small way that he or she could.

At the Salvation Army, donations of food and beverages spilled out onto the sidewalks. Sandwiches were sent to rescue workers with notes of encouragement, and hot, home-cooked meals were lovingly brought to firehouses. Spontaneous memorials sprang up all over the city as people silently gathered to share their grief and try to make sense of something beyond comprehension. The city came together to heal together. It felt as if we were one, that the city was a family. What was done to the few was done to the many, and all we could do was hold on to each other, giving our love and support.

Connections are made slowly; sometimes they grow underground.

—Marge Piercy

I had a compelling need to check on my friends in the city, on September 11—one by one. I headed to a friend's house to make sure that she and her husband were safe. The transit system was down and I found myself in an urgent mass of people coming up from Lower Manhattan. Among the throng I was surprised to find George, the maître d' of Milos, a restaurant in my neighborhood. It was such a relief to see someone I knew in the crowd. But George, normally vivacious and outgoing, was in shock. We both began talking, desperate to share our disbelief and horror. Suddenly, a stricken look came over George's face and he asked me if I would give him a hug. I didn't need to be asked twice. Our eyes brimming with tears, we wrapped our arms around each other, comforting and bolstering one another. "I knew there was a reason I walked down this street," he said, sighing.

My friends made all the difference to me at this time. I felt raw, vulnerable, disoriented. Yet each time someone reached out to me, it confirmed my faith in the goodness of people—even in the face of such a devastating and incomprehensible act. The generosity of my friends began the healing process for me. My family in Canada phoned every day to check in. Friends I hadn't heard from in years, from as far away as Europe, called to be sure that I was safe. My work team—Dominic, Shannon, and Regina—drew me into the safety of their families in New Jersey, as my own was so far away. Every call I received, every e-mail, warmed my heart and restored my sense of connection. I felt the care and concern of so many people enveloping me. Their loving strength provided stability and gave me something to hang on to after all had been so violently yanked away that September morning.

We don't live in a vacuum. If we think we can disconnect and not be affected, we are mistaken. It is vitally important for us to create a community that is nurturing and responsive, to contribute to that community, and to connect. If we don't we will have no well of love to drink from, no foundation of relationships from which to draw strength. Over time, without replenishment, we will eventually become isolated and alone. Without resources to fall back on, we cannot nurture ourselves fully. As wise women we now realize that our actions affect the community, and the community, in return, affects us. Our relationship with the community is connected like a circle with no end and no beginning. When we become part of that circle, we find our place. We feel that we belong, that we are part of a bigger story.

> We *always* need our family and our community ties to be strong. They are both the world we live in and our refuge from the world.

time after time

When we stay connected in the present—to family, friends, and community—we also connect to the past and the future. In this way we take our place in the chain of life that connects history to hope. We connect by reaching out where there is a need, by giving of our time, our energy, and our unique talents. We can reach out to our community by volunteering for clean-up programs, reading to children, or becoming companions to the elderly.

Every one of us, no matter who we are or what we do, has that power to make a difference and be remembered for it years later. George Bernard Shaw wrote, "Life is no brief candle to me. It is a sort of splendid torch which I have got hold of for the moment, and I want to make it burn as brightly as possible before handing it on to future generations." We all want to pass on what we have learned and experienced to our children and grandchildren, for generations to come. Staying connected also means connecting the generations. As wise women, we understand intuitively the need to create nurturing bonds between the generations, so that there is a richness, a depth, a usefulness and support that uplifts each generation. My dear friend Reece phrased it in a way that really moved me. He says he sees himself standing on the shoulders of his parents and his grandparents, and that bestows on him a sense of responsibility, as well as honor and humility for his own position in life.

We connect to all life that has come before us, and all life to come, when we consciously act as caretakers of all we have. I was struck by what Claude Lelouch said about his wonderful, sprawling farm perched on the cliffs of Normandy. Even as a young man he had an awareness that he was not the owner of his property, that he was "just caring for it until it passed on to the next owners," knowing that it would go on to the next generation, and the generation after that. His thoughtful words changed my view about owning anything *forever*.

spirit of place

Today we have so many impersonal chains dotting our landscape that many of us feel we've lost a sense of community. Well, something has been lost. What used to be such a large part of normal community life is now the exception for a great many people. I'm fortunate to have found a few places in my neighborhood where I can really feel connected. At one of my favorite neighborhood restaurants, Il Gattopardo, the chef, Vito, and the owner, Gianfranco, greeted me with such warmth and inclusion when I wandered into their restaurant for the first time that I just knew I had found a new home. Vito loves food, is proud of his cooking, and is full of life. In a matter of minutes he had me down in the kitchen, cooking pasta with the big, professional chef's machinery. We spent the entire afternoon cooking in the basement kitchen. He showed me how to form every shape of pumpkin ravioli, and to roll out spaghetti, linguine, and fettuccine from scratch—the Italian way. Then, he sent me home with a shopping bag filled with containers of pasta we had made together.

Vito is a little man from Italy who's cooked all over the Italian countryside. I am a small, Canadian girl living in New York City. On the surface we have nothing in common. And yet, we found a connection: a tremendous love for food, the making of food, the celebration of food—and a zest for life. I love Vito's aliveness, I love his joy, I love being around him!

Discovering Il Gattopardo helped me find more than a kindred spirit. The restaurant has become a neighborhood hub, a sort of community center. All my friends and I meet there regularly. It has become our place for business dinners, birthday parties, and company meetings. I've even worked on this book over Vito's excellent cuisine. That first warm and immediate welcome created a bond that has connected an entire community.

> *Surround yourself with people who respect and treat you well.*
> —CLAUDIA BLACK

Our gathering places—Il Gattopardo, Milos, the Garden Market, and Pane e Vino in Santa Barbara, and my favorite coffee hangout, Via Quadronno—maintain a sense of the past, a time when it was common to have a neighborhood restaurant open its arms to the local community and become a home away from home. For me, having a neighborhood restaurant that promotes relationships, knowing that there's somebody who is doing his or her part to build community ties by creating a warm, nurturing center in all our lives, fills me with appreciation and joy. Because of this feeling of community they have created we have a place to come together, to stay together, and to celebrate. It's important for all of us to find places where we can feel welcome, and I urge all of you to seek out and support places in your own neighborhood that create an atmosphere for people to come together. The venue doesn't have to be fancy just as long as you find a welcoming place to get together with friends and share. The local coffee shop can easily become a shared spiritual home if it's where you go to stay connected.

the butterfly effect

We have no idea of the impact we can have on other people's lives. The Chaos Theory, a branch of mathematics, has a principle called *the butterfly effect* that says you can't predict outcomes in nature, that a butterfly flapping its wings in Brazil can cause a tornado in Texas. Imagine that: the tiny flaps of a butterfly's wings could create minute disturbances in the atmosphere that grow and grow until they can affect entire weather patterns. Think of that seemingly insignificant smile, the one you flash to a perfect stranger. It can have the same effect. With one smile, you have a chance to elevate another person's mood in a second. You have created an opening for the person to pass on that positive feeling to another, and another, and another. Like the butterfly, you have started a chain reaction with limitless possibilities.

The effects of our actions may not be immediately clear to us, but the way we act always affects our environment and the people in it. A kind word or a thoughtful gesture can go farther than we know. Even something as seemingly insignificant as exchanging a

> *Life will bring you pain all by itself. Your responsibility is to create joy.*
> —MILTON ERICKSON

smile or holding a door open for someone can profoundly affect another person. In fact, wishing for someone's good, sending positive thoughts his or her way, praying for someone, *whether the person knows it or not*, can have a profoundly positive effect on his or her life. A study published in *The Archive of Internal Medicine* (10/25/99) showed that praying for patients, *even without their knowledge*, is linked to their improved health.

One day while in a taxi in New York City, I happened to ask the driver to roll up the window because it was getting a bit chilly. He became agitated, muttering angrily under his breath. Like any New Yorker, my first reaction was to ignore him. Then a sudden impulse changed my mind and I decided to press forward.

"Did it bother you that I asked you to roll up the window?"

He snapped back, "Of course it didn't bother me."

I persisted, "Well, it sounds like you've had a really rough day."

He responded that he had been having a really rough *year*. I asked him what had happened, and finding a friendly ear, he proceeded to tell me about the difficulties in his life. He *had* had a really rough year. His wife had been hospitalized and after a long, painful illness had passed away. He had lost a son as well and was struggling with finances when he was recently robbed. Now he was alone, trying to pick up the pieces of his life. By the time we reached my destination, he had finished his story. The simple and direct way he related his hardships moved me. Not really knowing how I could help, I offered him my sympathy for all he had experienced. He thanked me and we said good-bye. As I started to walk away, he remained there, leaning out his cab window, watching me go.

Suddenly, he called out, "Lady, will you do something for me?" I looked back at his open face, so earnest at that moment.

"If I can," I responded.

And cautiously, as though afraid of my response, he gently asked, "Will you pray for me?"

"Of course." Touched by the intimacy of the connection between us I responded without hesitation. It was a moment that was so simple, yet so human.

With a nod of satisfaction, as if a deal had been brokered between us, he drove off, leaving me stunned on the sidewalk staring as his cab disappeared in the distance. I knew I was holding a treasure in my heart. A moment so true, so real, had happened, *with a perfect stranger.* I realized that it was the decision to reach out and connect that allowed me to receive so much back in return. The giver is always the receiver.

We want to give. We want to connect. We want to do something extraordinary and make a difference. Often when we have that impulse we think we must be part of some grand, global effort: ending starvation in Sudan, wiping out AIDS in Africa, freeing women in Afghanistan. Each of these causes is urgent and worthwhile. But no kindness is wasted, no consideration is unimportant or frivolous, and the simple truth is that great changes can come from small and gentle acts. A hello to the cashier in your grocery store, a thank-you to a salesperson who waited on you, a wave to the newsstand vendor as you grab your daily paper—all these

> *Small things, done with great love, bring joy and peace.*
> —MOTHER TERESA

simple actions can have life-changing effects. These small, seemingly inconsequential acts can uplift and shift a person's view of life in an instant.

Life is made up of so many routine acts. But if we look at them in the right way we can turn the ordinary into the extraordinary. Just as my friend Hilton said in Nurture Your Spirit, "Any routine can be made special, depending on how you look at it. A day is made up of a thousand ordinary moments. It is up to us to make those moments extraordinary."

> **If we appeal to the best part of other people in the way we treat them, we will invariably be rewarded with their best.**

We need to remember that we are all connected, that caring acts can transform each one of us, and at the very least can put us back in touch with our heart—sometimes when we need it most. It's hard to reach midlife without having a low point, a time when you feel so depleted you think you won't be able to make it through the next moment. I reached my lowest point trying to maintain my equilibrium while striving to keep my daughter, Ryan, in college. My life at that time felt like an onslaught of trials. Every day was a struggle. It was taking every ounce of my energy and all my finances just to get by. The moment I would get through one obstacle, another would come rushing in to grab my attention.

Taking Ryan's little secondhand Volkswagen in to be repaired one day, I was devastated to find a fistful of her parking tickets hidden in the glove compartment. As if that weren't enough, the tickets were so delinquent that when the mechanic parked the car outside the repair shop, it was impounded almost immediately. I had to go from the shop, to the impound lot, to the police station, and then finally the DMV, where a long, winding line awaited me, snaking slowly up to the counter. As the hours ticked by I had the time to run all my troubles over and over in my head: my shortage of funds, my mounting debts, my daughter's carelessness, my seeming helplessness in life, my sense of isolation. I felt as if I were doing everything all alone. By the time I got to the window, tears were streaming down my face. I had given up. The woman behind the counter took one look at me and kindly handed me a Kleenex. With compassion and an encouraging smile she asked me what had happened. I ended up telling her the whole story.

She immediately went into action, assuring me that everything would work out. First, she directed the people behind me to another line; then she looked at the unpaid tickets and found she could cut the bill down. I don't quite know how she did it—I wonder to this day. But somehow this kind woman felt compassion for the person in front of her, the irrational, soggy woman, juggling Kleenexes and trying to attend to her runny, sniffling nose. It might have been a mistake (I'm not really sure), but I just remember that this dear, warm-hearted woman found a way for me to pay less. And as if that weren't enough, she also helped me with all the convoluted paperwork. I left the DMV rejuvenated. Uplifted by her kindness, her caring, and her thoughtfulness, I walked out a different person, a hopeful person. The warm connection she made with me changed my world. Suddenly I felt I could do it. I really could take care of things. I hoped. I trusted. I believed. And all because a stranger felt compassion and connection to another stranger.

blessed bonds

I have been blessed with a supportive family. As far back as I can remember my parents created a home that was—and still is—a haven. We lived very modestly as I was growing up, but my mother had a generous heart and always shared what we had with those who were less fortunate. When my sister Lynda went to live in England, her bedroom was offered to a series of troubled young girls who had no place to go. Living in such close quarters with these girls, I found that my teenage experiences became intertwined with the stories of the hardships they recounted. The contrast between their lives and what my family and I shared shocked me, and opened my eyes to the inconsistencies of the world.

By reaching out to help others, my parents set an example that I try to incorporate into all aspects of my life. When you feel you have been given a lot, as I feel my family has been given, then you want to give back to those who've had less. My parents have never refused anyone in need, and all of my siblings have had a profound effect on others and their community. While raising her own family, my younger sister, Darilyn, fought great odds to become a lawyer to help protect women who were oppressed. My younger brother, James, has an uncanny sensitivity for healing those in need. People constantly seek him out for advice. He always has the right word or the deep, insightful advice that uplifts their spirits, and he sends them on their way full of renewed confidence.

Every aspect of life becomes worthwhile when you can give of yourself.

My older sister, Lynda, has twins and is an active member of an organization for multiple births. Moved by the suffering of parents who had lost one or both of their twins, she fought for their acceptance into the organization—and won. "These babies *lived*, no matter how short a time," she says. "It's important that their lives are acknowledged." Lynda soon realized she had an ability to help those with losses to heal, so she took it a step further. She researched everything she could find about loss, enrolled in bereavement courses, and studied at hospitals. Today, fifteen years later, Lynda is the president of Multiple Births Canada. She writes a quarterly newsletter, *Forever Angels*, has her own Web site, and counsels hundreds of families worldwide on loss and bereavement. She recently won the National Canadian Volunteer Award for Bereavement. The letters of gratitude she receives sustains her: "When you give, you get. I just say to myself, one family at a time. These people are my inspiration."

Living your life as service is a noble endeavor. Everyone has something to give; we only have to recognize how we can serve. My parents took the lead and my brother and sisters followed. Loving and caring for people outside the family circle has made each one of us stronger, and today that love and support extends across the generations: from my parents and family, to me and to my daughter Ryan, and her children. Among us we create a loving circle—giving, receiving, and staying connected.

My relationships with my girlfriends form some of my strongest bonds. They are a foundation of strength and support for me, a source of tremendous laughter, sharing, and joy. Their love and friendship carry me through thick and thin. It's hard to go even a day without speaking to them. By listening to my friends' problems and helping them find solutions, I've learned so much more about the nature of life. We all have challenges to face, no matter who we are. Some people are better equipped to deal with these challenges than others, but everyone feels his or her own pain. As friends we have an unspoken agreement to support each other toward our own true self—almost a pact—and at times it takes bravery on each of our parts to say, "There's something not right. I think we need to talk." But what it always comes back to is that we know each of us has the other's best interests at heart. Each of us comes from a place of love, and each of us wants to see the other be true to herself, true to her dreams and accomplishments. When one of us succeeds, we all succeed. And of course, throughout all our experiences together, we share the same language—our laughter and our joy! Life—the good, the bad, *and* the ugly—is so much more meaningful when we share it with friends.

> *My glory was I had such friends.*
>
> —W. B. YEATS

clearing the air

We know when we are in sync with another person when we just feel good in another person's presence. This is staying connected at its best. But connections can be challenging at times, especially in our closest relationships. We may be asked to be patient, to be courageous, and to constantly renew our love, even when it is the most difficult for us.

There are many ways to bridge difficulties in our close relationships, and all families and friendships do have their challenges. It's important to find the means to navigate these obstacles. Who wants to keep dragging old hurts around with them like so many excess pounds? As women at midlife, one thing we know for sure is that we just don't want to waste the time, or the energy for that matter. Why carry around old wounds that get in the way of closeness with our family members and friends? It's a burden too heavy to carry.

Staying connected in relationships that have conflict doesn't have to involve major confrontations. If you're at an impasse with a family member or a friend, sometimes bridging the gap can be as simple as a quick phone call or e-mail to check in and say, "I was just thinking about you." In fact, using e-mail can be a particularly good way to stay in touch through family discord. You can let difficult matters settle, yet still stay connected and remind the person of your good intentions. An e-mail with a short positive message can often be the best and most painless way to approach a relationship until you, or the other person, are able to talk more directly.

Sometimes our personal relationships can become challenging simply because we are not up-to-date with each other's lives. When we don't know what's going on in someone's day-to-day life, we tend to imagine all sorts of things, especially in relation to ourselves. False ideas can build out of nothing, causing us to feel rifts where there may be none. At the very least, we can feel neglected or allow others to feel so. When we do disconnect, for whatever reason, there is no better way to heal than to make the attempt to stay in touch, regularly and sincerely, even when at times we feel like doing the opposite.

When things aren't harmonious, I try not to let too much time go by; I think the longer you let things go, the more difficult it is to repair the damage. The distance can grow

> *The past is never where you left it.*
> —KATHERINE ANNE PORTER

and grow over time, making it seem impossible to reconnect. When you reach out right away, or at an opportune moment, you can sometimes save years of buildup and misunderstanding. If you can't find the words and don't know what to say, try simply, "I'm thinking of you. I just want you to know I care." Or, "We don't have to agree, but I still love you and care about you." It doesn't matter whether you send a note, make a call, or shoot off a quick e-mail. What does matter is that you make the effort to make the connection.

Misunderstandings can arise between loved ones, so it's important to "keep clean" by voicing things. Obviously, we don't need to (and shouldn't) nitpick every little thing that comes up. As Ryan once said to me when I was fussing because, once again, she'd permanently stuck the soap to the soap dish in my shower, "Mom . . . pick your battles!" (What mother hasn't heard that one?)

If we react to every little perceived slight we are not moving our relationships forward. But we usually have a pretty good sense of what is important and what does need to be shared—we just have to use our judgment. When we don't voice what's wrong to those we are closest to, we create a little distance. And that distance will widen with time if it isn't taken care of. When we shove our voices down inside, ignoring them, we also disconnect from ourselves, shutting off from our wisdom and our true life. Staying connected requires that we remain honest with our loved ones. So, choose the right time to talk, and ask permission from the other person before you venture forth. In other words, we want to use our wisdom to be sensitive to others, as well as to take care of ourselves.

I learned this myself as an adult after a childhood of silly tiffs with my younger sister, Darilyn. Dari and I shared a bedroom growing up, so we had ages to build up sisterly differences; we didn't see eye-to-eye on many things. In fact, some relatives didn't even want to have us over together! Who knows what our path would have been if we'd stuck to our old

THE 5 PRINCIPLES OF AGELESS LIVING

ideas about each other? But out of the blue, one day at a health club when we were in our twenties, Dari genuinely reached out to me. She simply wanted to know what was going on in my life. To her surprise, the reality of my life was nothing like her picture of it. She thought her sister the model had a life that was all glamour and flashbulbs! But once we talked—*really* talked—she realized that my life wasn't as easy as she had thought. Things were definitely not as they appeared.

Because of that epiphany a door opened between us, and our relationship did a complete 180-degree turn. In that moment when she realized some of my difficulties, my sister became my supporter, my champion, my protector, *and* my friend. Now we are *very* close; we love sharing—sharing about being sisters, daughters, parents, and now new grand-mothers. One moment of truth in a lifetime of assumptions unwrapped a tremendous gift for both of us.

If Dari hadn't been interested or patient enough to lis-ten, if our conversation had never taken place, I might never have seen how true she really is, and how rich her accom-plishments are. She's a single mom raising three children and running a business, who put herself through college at night to become a lawyer. As if all that weren't enough, she now runs marathons! If Dari hadn't opened the door to the woman we each had become I would have gone right past a gold mine in my life. I would never have developed a true relationship with her. Today, I can say things to Dari that I can't say to anybody else, because once, long ago, we whispered in bed together late at night in the dark.

how to stay connected

Staying connected takes very little effort. The phone call or a quick note that says "I miss you," or even a simple "Thank you" speaks volumes. So does remembering birthdays and special occasions or even sending a small bouquet of flowers for no special reason. Once when my sister Dari was sick and feeling a little down, I happened to have the FTD florist catalog in front of me. Inside, it had flowers, "For a Sick Friend." It was a cozy bouquet with a little teddy bear, a special coffee mug and coffee, hot soup mix, and a little balloon. It was inexpensive and adorable and I couldn't resist. I picked up the phone, placed my order, and just a short while later, a deliveryman was standing on Dari's doorstep. What a difference it made to her day.

We can always find opportunities to connect and brighten someone's day if we put our minds to it. I think it's wonderful when, no matter how busy we are, we can still try to fold in personal touches in our contact with others. My friend Deb Shriver, who has a high-pressure PR job, always makes the time to dash off a handwritten card saying, "Let's get together, too much time has gone by." Carol Hamilton, with all her duties as President and General Manager of L'Oréal Paris, still remembers my birthday and special occasions with a handwritten note. Leonard Lauder at Estée Lauder is famous for taking the time to pen personal thank-you notes, as does my friend Dan Lufkin. I look forward to receiving the trademark penciled notes of thanks and goodwill that Dan finds the time to send, no matter how busy his schedule. My dear friend Donna Kail dashes me off delightful postcards from all her work trips around the country and another friend, Rusty Pierce, drops me notes with photos enclosed of her baby boy, so that I can stay connected. All these unexpected notes always make me feel uplifted.

My daughter, Ryan, writes beautiful notes of thoughts and thanks, all of which I treasure and save. And she always remembers I-love-you's. I still cherish a note she wrote me as a young child:

"Remember: You R the best mother in this <u>WORLD</u>."

(Now, what mom wouldn't appreciate a message like that?)

reach out and touch

My friend Regina was once trying to reach her mom, Vincenza, on the telephone, but the line was constantly busy. When she finally got through Regina said, "Mom, why were you on the phone so long? I've been trying and trying to get hold of you!" In a perfectly normal voice, her mother replied, "Honey, I was saving a life." Vincenza has very strong relationships with her girlfriends; they rely on her daily to talk them through their problems until they are resolved. For her friends, Vincenza really is a life saver!

We are so fortunate to live in a world where everyone is just a phone call or an e-mail away. We all have such busy lives that sometimes a short phone call really is the best and only way to maintain a steady connection. I make a habit of calling my mother each weekend, no matter where I am in the world. It makes such a difference for her—and for me. We both look forward to the calls. My daughter and I also communicate at least every few days. It would feel strange if we didn't. I talk with my girlfriends every day—*all* of them—at least once a day! Life would be a lot less fun without those calls.

> With great communication, in person or on the phone, you actually receive the person's positive energy, the person's *shakti,* and they yours. That's why it makes you feel so good. Being in touch with those we love, whenever we can, is vital to our sense of joy and happiness.

Reaching out can propel your relationships forward quickly, even with distance, years, and events between you. Staying connected keeps our relationships current. The phone can limit real intimacy, but then again I've worked out very complicated parts of relationships by phone when I've had to. (As wise women, we know how to use our resources!)

Time spent with loving, nurturing family and friends can refresh our relationships and prevent us from growing apart. By sharing new experiences with each other we create new memories. And this can be important whether we are forming new friendships or building relationships back up again. It's important to remember that we all evolve and change. It's important to know who someone has become and is still becoming, instead of staying fixed on who we thought they were. We can't stay connected and create new happy memories if our experiences of loved ones remain stuck in the past. We can't fully share our joys and continue on the path of life together if we stubbornly carry with us only the past. But we can be loving, nurturing family members and friends ourselves by staying open to others' growth and finding the opportunities to share our own.

The telephone and e-mail can connect us quickly to people, but sometimes we need to share more directly. Spending time with our loved ones in person can often seem logistically taxing when everyone is on the go, but it's important to make the time for these one-on-one visits to affirm our family's and friends' importance to us, and our importance to them. Don't wait for a formal occasion, a wedding or an anniversary, or God forbid, a funeral, to stay connected. Try not to say "We must get together soon," without adding *when*.

I know that whenever my friends and family come together, we all say, "We should get together more often." Let's make good on that.

create celebrations

One afternoon at my friend Elisabeth's magical farm, we decided to have a pasta contest among her many guests. As there were several Italians, winning would be a matter of national pride! It was exciting to see everyone take up the challenge. In every nook and cranny of her sprawling farmhouse, guests were busily creating their best pasta. Shouts and laughter and a sense of celebration came from every room, as did an amazing array of aromas. Finally, one by one, with great pride, the contestants displayed their pasta marvels.

> *Life isn't a matter of milestones but of moments.*
> —ROSE FITZGERALD KENNEDY

Each dish was better than the next, and as we all judged, very often the verdict was, "I'm not sure, I have to have just a little more." Finally, sated, we happily judged them all the best. It was a great excuse for a celebration!

Dream up your own reasons—or "excuses"—to celebrate and stay connected with people. You can create an occasion to celebrate almost anything: moving into a new home, the completion of a project, an impromptu visit from a friend. Celebrate May Day, the full moon, the summer solstice, a special anniversary—even your favorite chocolate cake. Or have no reason—besides being glad you are alive. To me, that is always reason to celebrate!

During my stay in an ashram in India, even though we were studying Eastern religion, we celebrated the special times of all religions. We rejoiced in the days of the moon coming out, the sunrise, the sunset, Christmas, Chanukah, saints' days, holy days. Every day was a special day. I realized then that that is the best way to live life—celebrate *each* day.

Just as we don't have to wait for an occasion, we shouldn't forget that even the usual occasions for celebrating can be made extraordinary with just a little bit of effort and imagination. My friend Christine and her husband, Armyan, alternate surprising each other on their anniversary each year. One year, when it was Armyan's turn, he lovingly "kidnaped" Christine and took her for a drive up the California coast without giving her any clues about where they were going. Eventually he turned onto a deserted dirt road and parked the car. Then Armyan led Christine, who was rather excited, to a secluded spot with a staggering view. A blanket was spread for a gorgeous picnic; he had thought of everything—chilled wine, her favorite foods, and a loving note. She said it was one of the most romantic anniversaries ever, one that would be very difficult to top.

come together

Living in Los Angeles, Christine knows that many people who end up there are a long way from home. To remind them of their family connections, Christine extends an open invitation for strays to come to her home for Sunday dinner—*any* Sunday. We all know we can wend our way to her house, without any advance notice, and share with her, her family, and other homeless friends, a yummy, home-cooked meal. These Sundays connect us. Her get-togethers are so loving, so intimate and welcoming, that everyone feels a sense of home away from home.

Each of us can organize events around people, and people around events. We can open our homes for charitable causes, we can form book clubs and other special-interest clubs for people to get together, or create welcome parties for out-of-towners. All it takes is a willingness to give. Sometimes, however, we really do have to be persistent. It took almost a year for me to get together with three of my wonderful friends: Deb, Mary Lou, and Carole. These busy women never seemed to be free at the same time. Mary Lou and Deb were in New York when Carole was in Los Angeles. When Carole returned, Deb had to leave on a business trip to South Africa. Then, just as we thought we were all finally going to meet, *I* was the cause of a last-minute change of plans. But everyone was persistent, and thanks to the scheduling finesse of Deb, we at last arranged our long-overdue dinner.

Inspired by a story that another friend had told me of an amazing gathering she had organized, I asked each of my friends to bring along to dinner a small object that held special meaning, something she could share with the rest of the group. The evening was wonderful from the start—filled with laughter, shared secrets, and stories—even before we revealed our personal objects. And then, one by one, we offered our treasures and stories to the group. Mary Lou was first. She tenderly pulled out a small object from her bag and set it on the table. It was a little castle that she had carried around for twenty years, a little castle that constantly reminds her that anything is possible, that all her dreams really can come true. Deb was next. Presenting a photograph of her husband and her dog, she stated simply and strongly that "everything I love is in this picture." Carole left her object at the office (she was running late!), but described to us her beautiful little frog, a talisman that she uses to recall the leap of faith that has brought her so far. And my offering? Well, since our long-overdue dinner landed on the Indian New Year, I brought with me Lakshmi, the Indian goddess of abundance and good fortune. Tradition tells us that our choice of New Year companions is auspicious. And as Lakshmi herself is the symbol of the New Year, a representation of inherent blessings, how could I not bring her with me, to share with my friends what I wanted for us all.

The evening was a tremendous success. Each woman told her tale so simply, so directly, and so profoundly that there was a hush as we all leaned in to listen. So much was said through each story, so much was revealed, that we felt closer to each other that night than I think we ever had. We cherished the shared experience of the evening, and were touched by the depth and eloquence of each woman and her willingness to reach out to her friends. Merely by using an object that had personal meaning, we strengthened our bond and went farther in our friendships than we had before. And before we all left to go home, we vowed not to let so much time pass before getting together again.

do something you love—for others

My mother never had a doll when she was little. She was well into her seventies before she decided to make up for lost time. Starting from scratch, she decided to take up the hobby of doll making, learning about the materials and molding and decorating techniques as she went along. She spent days *and* nights, blissfully immersed in her new passion. It takes hours and hours and hours to make a single doll, but when she's made it and painted it and fired it and dressed it—she gives it away! She does that, she says, just because it makes her feel good.

My mom works in a hospital and gives her dolls, crafted with such joy, to the sick children, who fall in love with them. When she offers them, she says, "It just gives me a good feeling when I see the look on a child's face—their eyes widen in amazement when they realize the doll is for *them*. That's worth every minute I spend making each one."

We all have pastimes we love. What could be better than to combine doing what we love with giving to others? When we do, we connect with people by offering them a part of our own joy. Our passions can serve real needs in our community: gardening in neglected neighborhoods, caring for animals in shelters, cooking for the homeless. Our efforts may not be necessary; they may simply be very much appreciated. Our passions can connect us, and then help us stay connected.

pay it forward

Volunteering is magic. You only have to do it once to receive an abundance of gifts in return. When we volunteer, we pass on to others what has been given to us. Volunteering not only connects us to new people, it help us link up to the entire community. In the Okinawan *yuimaru* tradition, each giver in the circle becomes a receiver, and each receiver a giver, all vital to the greater good.

One Maryland woman I once met, Jan, has lost more than twenty family members and friends to cancer. Instead of being totally devastated, she found a way to turn her pain into something positive. Creating a mountain retreat for children with cancer and their families, she gave them a place to be "normal" and have fun. Often, she dresses up as a clown, thrilling the sick children. On top of it, she makes it a point to find ways to grant them their wishes. One little girl with leukemia wished and wished for the chance to go to a wedding; Jan made her the flower girl at her *own* wedding!

My dear friend Michele is an intuitive who does healing work at her center in New York. She is often asked to hurry to someone's hospital bedside, when regular medical procedures have gone as far as they can. She has had amazing results working with patients with extreme illnesses. Michele is a remarkable person and someone I deeply admire. She continually volunteers her services, because, she says, "It's an opportunity to give what *I* have been given. It's a moment of intense truth where the possibility of miracles can happen. It's also the meeting place where giving and receiving become one. Sometimes I can't tell who is healing whom."

My friend John started an inner-city education program in Northern California called Making Waves. At-risk fifth graders who would never have had a chance to go to college are mentored and tutored all the way up through university. In less than fifteen years, John has been personally involved in the lives of over four hundred students. And every spring he attends at least twenty-five graduations. John started Making Waves simply because he wanted to make a difference. And he has literally changed the life of every child he has met.

Volunteering is moving from me to we!

We can all take action to connect with someone who needs us. Opportunities to volunteer are as close as our phone book or computer; hospitals, shelters, churches, and charities are some of the places we can start. Organizations that truly make a difference such as Points of Light, Make-A-Wish, One-to-One, and your local Volunteer Center (see Resource Guide) will help you get started—and will welcome your enthusiasm.

community chest

Every community needs some help; we need only to find out how we can help our own. Neighborhood cleanups, school improvement, sprucing up parks and playgrounds—there are as many ways to make a difference as there are volunteers. A group of my friends discovered one impoverished community that always welcomes our helping hand. We regularly come together to help clean up and plant new trees. The residents appreciate it; it's uplifting to know we've helped, and the community does look better.

You don't have to organize anything (though it's great if you can); what's important is your participation. There is always a drive to collect something. Look for notices on supermarket and store bulletin boards, in community newspapers, at churches, synagogues, and mosques—even if you're not a member—at schools, the dry cleaners, wherever people congregate. Donate clothes, canned goods, toiletries, toys, even used eyeglasses. I have found that someone will be grateful—even thrilled—for every item. (If you have any doubt about that, look at eBay on the Internet.) Everyone has something to offer. And I truly believe that, deep down, we all *want* to contribute.

> *What we must decide is perhaps how we are valuable, rather than how valuable we are.*
> —Edgar Z. Friedenber

not so trivial pursuits

We can connect with people who share our interests by seeking out what interests *us*. We may be surprised to find what is available in our own community: lectures, classes, food or wine tastings, street fairs, reading clubs, film festivals, crafts and flower shows, antiques fairs, and even garage sales. Joining neighborhood associations is also a great way to connect with people.

A large city can feel like a cozy, small community when we meet new people and share pursuits. In New York, the 92nd Street Y offers some of the most fascinating lectures, from Itzak Perlman to Barbara Walters, from politicians to poets. When I am in Toronto, where my family lives, I like to join my father at his classes at the Y, where he faithfully goes every Sunday, keeping up his community connections.

I traveled to a yoga conference in Florida after seeing an announcement in the *Yoga Journal,* a magazine I love. I was taught by many of the great yoga teachers, from Rodney Yee to Baron Baptiste, and Shiva Ray to Rod Stryker. In one weekend, I met the whole yoga community. I also made new friends—women who came from all over the country to do something we all loved, together. That's where I began my wonderful friendship with yoga teachers Ila and Garrett Sarley, which continues to this day.

Magazines like *Yoga Journal* or *O: The Oprah Magazine, Health, Redbook,* and *Good Housekeeping,* publicize national events in your area. *More Magazine* promotes a yearly modeling contest for women aged forty and over. I was a judge at the very first one, and it brought amazingly interesting and powerful women from all over the country to New York City. It changed many lives.

We just have to make the effort to find opportunities for connection, from neighborhood "shopper" newspapers to brochures we can pick up in supermarkets. (I actually found a fascinating women's health conference going on in Santa Barbara this way.) If you can't find what you want, organize it. You can recognize ageless talent in your community by putting together an art show, holding a music recital, or starting a club. Use the community bulletin boards in bookstores, markets, and restaurants. Remember the movie *Field of Dreams?* In my experience, "If you post it, they will come."

Support school plays and drives. Some of the most fun I had as a child was participating in my community's annual garden event; we exhibited flowers and vegetables from our family garden and it was exciting to win ribbons for the things we had grown. Visit state fairs, 4-H Club events, rodeos, and sporting events. All these connect us to our community by making us feel the excitement of being part of a group. That's why we often prefer to watch a movie in a movie theater instead of on video—the group experience heightens the story for us.

We can find surprising opportunities for connection in unexpected places. My daughter, Ryan, wanted to learn needlepoint, so together we visited a small local crafts store in Brentwood, California, and lo and behold, there was a group of women gathered to teach each other the arts of needle-point and knitting!

Many of *us* have wisdom to pass along. If you have an interesting pursuit, why not let young people learn from you.

birthdays

I LOVE BIRTHDAYS! Mine and everyone else's. I love every opportunity to celebrate, but birthdays are *really* special. As a matter of fact, I signal my birthday months ahead (by the way, it's May 26!), and I've been known to have as many as three parties—or more, if I can cram another one in. I get so excited about my birthday parties that it gets everybody else excited. It's now become the norm that I will have *four* birth-day parties a year!

Why do I love birthdays so much? Because, every one is a chance to get together with friends, to love and celebrate each other. I adore the birthday traditions: the cake, the candles, the blowing out of the candles, the good wishes, the presents.

This year, I did something different. I was visiting with Ryan and her husband, Christian, in Los Angeles on my birthday, and my closest friends were back in New York. So I decided to invite several friends from my younger years in L.A. to a small party. It was a wonderful opportunity for all of us to reconnect. At dinner, I had the extraordinary experience of going around the table and telling each person, one by one, why he or she was so special to me—and thanking the person for being my friend. There was a lot of laughter and tears.

My birthday was so poignant, I did it *again*—in New York. (Different group of friends.) And Ryan and Christian ended up being at *both* parties. This time, I wanted to bring out the silliness and the "little girl" in my friends. Ryan and I hit the Disney Store. Each of my girlfriends got a pink or blue feathered tiara; lots of stylish plastic jewelry in pastel colors; figurines of Snow White, Cinderella, and Belle from *Beauty and the Beast;* plastic cups with fairy-tale princesses on them; and small beaded purses. It was a little girl's party for big girls. And of course, it was held at our favorite restaurant, Il Gattopardo.

I also love giving birthday parties for my friends. I threw a surprise party at New York's Culinary Institute for my friend Reece. I told him I'd discovered this fabulous restaurant, located in an office building that no one knew about. He had no idea where I was taking him. Inside, he was completely surprised to find a dozen friends waiting in chef's aprons, surrounded by balloons, and ready to cook. With two chefs guiding us, we spent the evening cooking our own delicious dinner, and then we all sat down to feast.

We can make birthdays special with more than candles. Bake a cake from scratch for someone—perhaps their favorite double chocolate. Throw the party yourself; what better way to introduce all your friends and family to each other? Show your children and grandchildren that birthdays are just as special and important for grown-ups as they are for children. Make mountainous events out of birthday milestones; my father turned eighty this year and *every* Haddon family relative was there to surprise him!

> *Our birthdays are feathers in the broad wings of time.*
> —JEAN PAUL RICHTEE

Be creative in celebrating birthdays. Make up your own way to honor the birthday boy or girl, and resist the voice that says "I'm too old for birthdays." Why would we *not* want to celebrate our birthdays? Embrace these wonderful days that mark one more year of being *alive*. One more year of life and the *first* day of our own new year— what could be more joyous than that?

reunions

Reunions keep us connected with people who were meaningful in our past. When I was working in Montreal, I tried to reconnect with my schoolmates, to no avail. Then, planning a class reunion, a few classmates found *me* through the Internet and soon we were all using e-mail to search for our favorite old pals. I couldn't find my high school boyfriend, Bobby, but I did find my two best girlfriends: Joanie, who is living in Ontario with two children, and Susie, now on Canada's west coast, also a mom. There is a sense of touching deep roots when we reconnect with old friends, even if we've gone in completely different directions.

It is worth a little time and research to reconnect, to remember where you came from, and to honor that time. Our childhood friends are the ones who knew us when . . . when we were filled with all our hopes and dreams for the future.

Reunions celebrate where you came from, where you are today, and all that it took for you to get there. But reunions don't have to mean only *school* reunions. Organize a get-together for your own group of special friends, pals from camp, or even long-ago work colleagues. One friend, now in her mid-forties, gets together at least once every five years with her three best friends from childhood; they come together no matter what, from upstate New York, Denver, Cleveland and Washington, D.C., leaving husbands, boyfriends, and children behind for a girls' weekend.

If you have ever wondered, "Whatever happened to . . . ? I really *liked* her . . ." then you are opening a door to magic.

take a hike

I have hiked with my dad and my sisters, Lynda and Dari, since we were little. It was always with great excitement that we packed a lunch and challenged a mountain. (Actually, it was more like a steep hill, but it seemed mountainous to me then.) I continue to hike whenever I can. It's fun to discover a new area, through different trails, while enjoying nature and getting a good workout—*and* to be able to share the adventure with a family member or friend. Getting together outdoors without the distractions of our daily lives gives us the freedom to enjoy our personal connections. Sometimes when we are "out of context" we can really open up and strengthen our connections. I often hike with a friend, with my daughter, or even with my dad, so we have time to catch up. It's a great opportunity to bond and share a real sense of achievement.

Hiking is something we can do easily into our fifties, sixties, and beyond. And there are all levels of hikes, one for everyone. My father was the *oldest* person to climb Gros Morne Mountain in Newfoundland—he was in his late seventies at the time! Not only did it give him a thrilling triumph, he became closer to his hiking companion, my sister Lynda's adventurous husband, Arthur. Now, each year, my dad and Arthur share a challenge that uplifts them both and strengthens their family bond.

Family outings can create opportunities to spend time together in lighthearted ways. They lift us out of old family patterns, allowing us to create new, fresh memories and solidify the love we know is there. So . . . take a hike!

random acts of kindness

We all have opportunities to be an angel, moments when we can give spontaneously and make a difference in someone's life. You can donate your frequent flyer miles to those in need who are traveling for certain medical treatments. You can send an inner-city child to a Fresh Air camp. You can even provide donations to veterans' groups to help them stay connected. There are *so* many kind things we can do: giving gifts of long-distance calling cards, writing letters for those who can't write themselves, checking in on home-alones.

Each year when I was growing up, my family made a point of giving during the holiday season. At Christmastime, we would put a box together to send to less fortunate children. To this day, I remember giving up my Campbell's Soup doll and the feeling it gave me to know another child would delight in something I loved so much. It was hard to do, but that made saying good-bye to her all the sweeter. At a young age, it made me understand sharing, on a deeper level.

Wonderful things happen from simple acts of giving. A famous author I know and admire makes it a point to give anonymously, sometimes impulsively, whenever she sees a need. One day, while she was getting a manicure, she overheard a woman crying, pouring out her story in a foreign language. Concerned, my friend discreetly asked one of the manicurists what was wrong. She found out that the distraught woman's brother was dying of cancer and she and another family member couldn't afford to fly to him to say their last good-byes. The author went into action: using the nail salon as a liaison, she secretly delivered two round-trip tickets, so that the woman could be there for her brother. To this day, the awestruck lady knows only that a miracle happened. She has no idea who her angel was.

Be an angel! Do it because you can. Pay the toll of the car behind you. Pick up litter (yours, of course, as well as others'). You can buy lemonade from a child's stand, give a busy mother a break, bake cookies for someone who is homebound, or carry packages for seniors. My friend Michele's husband, Dillon, will put money in parking meters anonymously if he notices that they're about to expire. Another friend now carries jumper cables in her car because a stranger once revived her car's dead battery, just in case she can return the favor.

Staying connected is a way of sharing not only what we have, but also who we are. When we connect we become part of the whole, part of the divine plan. Our role then, however small, becomes more significant, and it is even more important for each of us to do our very best.

To give our best, we must live our best life. When we take care of ourself—look our best, nurture our spirit, discover our wisdom, and honor our body—we are living our best life, we are living true.

Gratitude unlocks the fullness of life. It turns what we have into enough and more.

—MELODY BEATTIE

The Adventure
Continues . . .

T oday, I am in my fifties, pursuing adventures that support my passions. ("Ventures," my three-year-old grandson calls them!) I am relishing the role of grandmother,
proud to be a pioneer exploring what it is that a grandmother
at midlife can look like—and *feel* like—today. Like most
women of my generation, I'm making it up as I go along. I do
the things I need to do for myself so that I have the excitement and energy to keep up with my delightful grandson,
Jaden, and my lovable granddaughter, Eliana. I hope to be able
to pass on to them any wisdom I may have garnered over the
years, and be open enough to share their bright viewpoints. In
short, in my fifties, I am on a new adventure.

This is the best time of my life so far. Today, I have
the joy of seeing my daughter grow, find love, and be a mom.
I am thrilled to watch from this unique vantage point, to

see a new, exciting chapter open for both her and for me. It's taken this long to put my arms around what I think is the best of me, and I'm looking forward to investigating it, experiencing it, and offering it in the years to come. It all looks good from here.

I am excited to know all the women I'm going to become. I'm eager to meet the person I will be at sixty, and seventy, and eighty. I want to be able to enter those years full of health, vitality, and optimism for what lies ahead. I believe in the grace and strength that come with age. I believe that with age comes a meeting of power and womanhood, and that's why I believe it is so important to practice the Ageless Living Principles to use them to find the amazing, brilliant, energetic, spirited, effervescent woman who lives in all of us—the woman we already are.

It takes a bit of courage, a bit of faith, and the desire to grow, but when we use the Ageless Living Principles to live consciously, we begin to see how our life can change. We can see how we gain freedom because we feel we look our best; how we are supported because we nurture our spirit; how we are secure because we have discovered our wisdom; and how strong we are because we honor our body. We become true. And, being true to life, we extend that truth to others by staying connected.

As women at midlife, we are compassionate, powerful, creative, wise beings, using the raw material that is our life to shape our growth and enhance our pleasure. However we get to our true life, we do arrive. Our perspective does shift. Our challenges may be personal, but the inner pull to reach our true potential and to live our fullest life is shared by all women. I believe that midlife is the stage of women's lives where our focus shifts from "What can I get out of life?" to a more meaningful "What can I become?"

We can all be graceful with aging. We can be light-hearted with our years. We can be joyful each day that we're here, alive, and participating. What we are striving for is to make graceful transitions at each stage, and to discover the gifts that every age has to offer us, if we're open to them. Know that we will have the courage and fortitude to face whatever is ahead of us. Know that whatever we *have* to go through, we *can* go through. We're in it for life! We might not have all the answers now, or ever, but we don't need to. We do our best. We can make the journey as interesting and enjoyable as possible, even as we uncover new answers—and new questions—along the way. The choice is ours. If the present

The great thing about getting older is that you don't lose all the other ages you've been.
—MADELEINE L'ENGLE

poses a hurdle or a challenge, the best way to go through it is simply to put one foot in front of the other, and go forward.

We have to be our own role models. My deepest wish is that you will embrace the Ageless Living Principles, use them daily in your lives and become the role models for those around you. Be the role model for your partner, for your daughter, even for your son. Be the role model for your friends and family, and for your community. But most of all, be the role model for yourself.

We may have a few more wrinkles, and a few more gray hairs, and it might take a bit more effort to get out of bed in the morning, but I wouldn't trade the wisdom, humor, and compassion that I have now just for a different date on my driver's license.

When my husband died, I doubted that I would ever think or say these things. Today, I love being a grandmother, running through the sprinklers with my grandson, as I did recently at my dad's eightieth birthday. And I love having coffee with my friends, and sharing in their lives. I look in the mirror and I like seeing myself as a woman in my fifties. I work out in the park and realize that although I can't quite do what I could at thirty, I still can do a heck of a lot.

I have enjoyed it all: the ups and the downs. I feel very lucky and grateful for what I do have in my life. I feel my life is full. All of us have the opportunity to live a full, fabulous life in our forties, fifties, sixties, and beyond. My greatest hope is that the Ageless Living Principles will help propel you on *your* journey toward your true life.

At midlife, we *are* ready. We are ready to live fully. Let's celebrate! *Grab* your life, hug it tightly to you, and run with it—*be* the woman you can be. Be the woman you *are* now!

> *You must do the thing you think you cannot do.*
>
> —ELEANOR ROOSEVELT

The Adventure Continues . . .

Ageless Living Dialogue

Q: What is the single most important thing a woman over
forty should know?

A: Your life is your own. It is what *you* make of it. We should
remember that a life is an arc. It has a beginning, a middle,
and an end. And *all* of our life is important. It is just common
sense that no one part can be more valuable than another.
Remember that life is a gift, and every day we have an opportunity to accomplish something meaningful for ourself and
for others. We need only to start with small changes to make a
big difference. It is our positive attitude that transforms a
good life into a great one.

Q: I'm trying hard to feel inspired about midlife, but hon-
estly, I just feel tired.

A: We are bombarded relentlessly by what we have to do all
day. No wonder we're always feeling so worn out. We have to

rejuvenate ourselves. We can't keep going back to the well and wondering why it finally ends up dry. We need to find ways to fill ourself back up, to take time for ourselves—quiet time—so that we can tune in to our inner voice. Often we become tired because we are not listening, because our inner voice isn't being heard. When life is reduced to just problem solving, then we have no way to plug into the magic that makes life joyous and we very quickly end up becoming exhausted. We need to take time in nature, time to share with those close to us, to be of service, and to follow what brings us into balance. When we do take time for ourself—it can be something as simple as taking a bubble bath—we feel rejuvenated and revitalized. We become inspired and are able to bring back enthusiasm into our daily life.

Q: Your advice to "look your best" is all very well—but you're a model. I look like most of the fifty-year-old women wandering the shopping malls. I haven't a chance of looking like you.
A: When you take the best care of yourself, when you want to look your best, you want to look your *own* best, not somebody else's. There will always be somebody who has a cuter nose, a flatter tummy, or more luxurious hair. We have to focus on what *we* have. When we present our best self, we feel confident. Then we are able to offer what we really have to give. At

midlife, with all the wisdom we've garnered over the years, we are in an extraordinary position to choose for the future ahead. By using the Ageless Principles as a guide, you can look your best no matter what your age.

Q: I've just turned fifty and wonder if I should start lying about my age?

A: You don't have to be bound by your age, but why deny such an essential part of who you are? Own your experience—and your age too.

Q: When I was younger, men used to whistle at me and I'd hate it. Now I miss it!

A: It's always great to have a little outward attention, confirmation that we look good. Every woman enjoys a compliment no matter what her age, but it's even better when we know it ourselves. When you take the time to look your best, it gives you the confidence to dare to do so many other things. With the wisdom of midlife, you have choices open to you to live a bigger life. If you take care of yourself, you create the energy and the vitality to do what you really want to do. Then you radiate the joy of life that does make heads turn. And, that is true beauty.

Q: I find that now I'm getting older I regret so many of the things I haven't done. I can't go back in time, so what can I do?

A: It's never too late to begin. One of my best friends went back to college to get her degree while in her mid-forties. Another friend quit the "perfect" job to do something that her heart directed her to do, while she too was in her mid-forties. We just need to know that midlife is the gateway to begin the second half of our life, with the added bonus of having a bank of wisdom at our disposal. We can travel, we can learn a new language, we can take cooking classes, pottery classes, even jewelry classes. There are so many courses and classes available to us. It just takes the energy and enthusiasm to know it's possible. Why would we want to go back in time when there's so much ahead of us!

Q: I believe that I'm an attractive woman, but it's hard to hold my head high when everything I see tells me that looking good is the same as looking young.

A: Our generation makes up a third of the population in this country. We're 43 million women strong. We are one of the most powerful demographics in this country. Remember that! The advertising, media, and beauty industries are only just beginning to catch up with this kind of power. As a group, we women are the ones who are going to change the way the media portray us in midlife. But first, we have to change the way *we* think about ourselves. We need to connect to the wisdom that we have and remind ourselves of the value of *who* we are now and what we have to offer. At midlife, we are looking for real meaning and in that search the answers will come. We do that by taking care of ourselves: by eating right, by looking our best, by cherishing our experiences, by adding to our wisdom, and by reaching out to others. So hold your head up high. This is your time. As my friend Carole's grandmother always says "Feel good, look good. Look good, do good."

Q: Finding the time to take care of myself is almost impossible to fit in during a day. How do I find the time to do things for myself with all the other demands on my day?
A: Who nurtures the nurturer? The only one who can is you. You must set aside a certain amount of time during the day that is your time, a time when you can become calm, commune with nature, and listen to your inner voice. You need to be able to rejuvenate so that you can do all the things you need to do in a day. It is imperative that you find simple ways to increase your inner joy and weave them into your life so that it becomes a part of it. You can set aside a sticky note that reminds you it's time to go for a walk, to breathe, to meditate, or make a standing appointment with a girlfriend to share a

walk in the park. Keep a journal by your bed and set aside time to write in it. Make time to meditate by setting your alarm a bit earlier. There are so many ways to rejuvenate, and by peppering appointments for yourself throughout your day, you'll find you have the energy to get through all you have to do, *and* feel energized.

Q: Midlife may be a time of new challenges, but it also brings new—and huge—responsibilities; for instance, caretaking for aging and ill parents. How can women navigate these very real issues that so many of us face, and still have energy, optimism, time, and money left over for ourselves?
A: We do, each one of us, have responsibilities that we must face and these are very real. Yet, if we don't have the personal resources to take care of these responsibilities, then where do we end up? It is important that we properly take care of ourselves so that we are able to give what needs to be given. That means getting the proper rest, eating well, exercising regularly, and spending some time in developing inner strength. Then we will always have resources to fall back on.

Q: How can a woman see and appreciate what she truly has?
A: Gratitude affects attitude. Gratitude for what we have is one of the single most powerful feelings around. It can turn ordi-

nary moments into extraordinary ones. The feeling of gratitude can heighten our appreciation for what we already have, no matter how little it may be. One way to practice gratitude is to keep a gratitude journal by your bedside. Look back at the end of the day and make a list of all the things you are grateful for. You may be surprised by how long your list may be.

Q: What's the single most important thing a woman at midlife can do to change her life for the better?

A: Realize that every day is a gift, an opportunity for adding meaning. Understand that no experience is without value, that there have been no wasted moments. No matter what has happened to you in your life, know that it is the way you look at your experiences that gives them value. There is a treasure in every challenge and it is up to each one of us to find it. It's all in your attitude. That's what makes you wake up in the morning and say to yourself, "Today is the first day of my life. It's an adventure. What will happen next?"

Q: What do you think about cosmetic surgery to help "look your best"?

A: Cosmetic surgery is a personal choice, but I would recommend that women look at the natural alternatives that are available first. It's good to ask yourself *why* you are having cosmetic surgery. Is it for you or to please someone else? It's also important to remember to focus on what you have gained over time, not what you have lost.

Q: I work with a lot of young people who think it's clever to refer to me as "a woman of a certain age." I hate it!

A: Tell them they've got it wrong: you're not a woman of a certain age, you're a woman of certainty!

Midlife Myths and Maxims

MYTHS	MAXIMS
Physical and mental vitality are somehow tied to women's most fertile years.	Looking great means looking great—not looking *great for your age*.
The appearance of aging is inevitable—dull hair and skin, wrinkles, sagging . . .	There is something to be grateful for in every moment.
How a woman looks reveals her age.	We show what we wear, but we model what we are.
A woman's life is over after forty—or if not, it's in decline.	We have more to give now than we ever have, *if* we choose to nurture and give it.
As a woman ages she is limited in her abilities and activities.	
Menopause signals the end of a woman's best years.	Women at midlife have the confidence to demonstrate their personal style.
Dressing appropriately at midlife means conservative, read *dowdy*.	When we go within, we never go without.
	Substance only enhances style.
Relationships at midlife are based on nostalgia and shared experiences earlier in life, and it's unlikely we will establish new, deep ties.	We *can* move through and beyond midlife with grace, beauty, and joy.
	We *can* make new, deep friendships at every age.
Having spirituality in our life shows a fear of mortality.	Beauty is not the sole province of the young.
Women over fifty become invisible—it's inevitable.	Spirituality is our trust that all is good, no matter how things appear.

Resource Guide

the adventure

Just Ask a Woman is a strategic marketing company that understands that women control the purse strings—www.justaska woman.com; 79 Madison Avenue, 12th floor, New York, NY 10016; 212-725-8251

principle 1: look your best

skin

DERMATOLOGISTS:

Dr. Lydia Evans—consulting dermatologist to L'Oréal Paris, with a private practice at 229 King St., Chappaqua, NY 10514; 914-238-1500

Dr. Amy Lewis—120 E. 75th St., New York, NY 10021; 212-288-6133

Dr. Suzan Obagi—Cosmetic Surgery and Skin Health Center Blaymore II, Suite 103, 1603 Carmody Court, Sewickley, PA 15143; 724-940-7546

Dr. Katie Rodan and Dr. Kathy Fields—www.rodanandfields.com; 6114 La Salle Ave., Box 442, Oakland, CA 94611; 888-995-5656

To find a dermatologist in your area, visit the American Academy of Dermatology website, www.aad.org/findaderm_intro.html

CLEANSERS AND TONERS:

Neutrogena Extra Gentle Cleansing Bar—www.neutrogena.com; 800-582-4048; available at drugstores

Neutrogena Maximum Strength
Oil-Controlling Cleansing Pads—
www.neutrogena.com;
800-582-4048; available at
drugstores

UpStage cleansing sponges—
available at drugstores

NOURISHING
PRODUCTS:

Aveeno Clear Complexion Daily
Moisturizer—www.aveeno.com;
877-298-2525; available at
drugstores

Catrix 5 Correction Cream—
www.catrix.com; available from
dermatologists

Catrix Rosacea Therapy—
www.catrix.com; available from
dermatologists

Clé de Peau Beauté Emulsion
Protectrice Tendre—
www.cledepeau.com;
info@cledepeau.com

Clé de Peau Beauté Essence
Appaisante—www.cledepeau.com;
info@cledepeau.com

Clé de Peau Beauté
Masque Transparence—
www.cledepeau.com;
info@cledepeau.com

Clinique Moisture On-Call—
www.clinique.com; 800-419-4041

Crème de la Mer Moisturizing
Lotion—available at upscale
department stores

Estée Lauder Advanced Night
Repair—www.esteelauder.com;
877-311-3883

Estée Lauder Daywear Protective
Anti-Oxidant Crème SPF 15—
www.esteelauder.com; 877-311-3883

Eucerin Protective Moisture Lotion
SPF 25—www.eucerinus.com;
available at drugstores

GlyTone Sulphur Masque—
available from dermatologists

Joey New York Calm & Correct
Gentle Soothing Moisturizer—
www.sephora.com; 877-SEPHORA;
available at Sephora stores

Kiehl's Sodium PCA Oil-Free
Moisturizer—www.kiehls.com;
800-KIEHLS-2

Lancôme—www.lancome-usa.com; 800-LANCOME:

Absolute Replenishing Cream SPF 15
Acné Contrôle Daily Acne Medication Gel-Cream
Hydra Contrôle Mat
Hydra-Intense Masque
Primordiale Intense
Re-Surface Retinol Concentrate Wrinkle Corrector—Day & Night
Vitabolic Deep Radiance Booster

La Roche-Posay Effidrate—www.laroche-posay.us; available from dermatologists

La Roche-Posay Toleriane Soothing Protective Light Facial Fluid—www.laroche-posay.us; available from dermatologists

L'Oréal Paris—www.lorealparisusa.com; available at drugstores:

Age Perfect Day Cream
Age Perfect Night Cream
FUTUR.e Moisturizer Normal to Oily
Pure Zone Skin Relief Oil-Free Moisturizer
Revitalift

Medicis Lustra—Medicis Pharmaceutical; 602-808-8800; available from dermatologists

Neutrogena Moisture for Sensitive Skin—www.neutrogena.com; 800-582-4048; available at drugstores

Oil of Olay Sensitive Skin Active Hydrating Fluid—www.olay.com; available at drugstores

Orlane B21 Crème Fluidratante—www.orlaneparis.com

Shiseido Future Solution Total Revitalizing Cream—www.sca.shiseido.com; available at department stores

Shiseido Pureness Matifying Moisturizer Oil-Free—www.sca.shiseido.com; available at department stores

Shiseido Pureness Moisturizing Gel-Cream—www.sca.shiseido.com; available at department stores

Topix Replenix Green Tea Cream—available from dermatologists

Tri-Luma Cream—
www.triluma.com; available from
dermatologists

PROTECTION:

Coppertone SPF 30 Oil Free
Faces—www.coppertone.com;
available at drugstores

Crème de la Mer sunblock—
available at upscale department
stores

La Roche-Posay Anthélios 60—
available from dermatologists

Mustela Total Sun Protection
Stick—www.sephora.com;
877-SEPHORA; available at
Sephora stores

Natura Bissé sunblock—
www.naturabisse.es; 800-7NATURA

Neutrogena UVA/UVB Sunblock
Lotion SPF 45—
www.neutrogena.com;
800-582-4048; available at
drugstores

Orlane B21 Crème Fluidratante—
www.orlaneparis.com

Rit Sun Guard Laundry
Treatment—www.ritdye.com;
available at drugstores

Sea & Ski Advanced Sunblock
Lotion SPF 50; available at
drugstores

Shiseido Sunblock Face Cream
SPF 35—www.sca.shiseido.com;
available at department stores

SPECIALTY
PRODUCTS:

Proactiv Solution—
www.proactiv.com;
800-950-4695

Retin-A—www.retinamicro.com;
800-426-7762; available from
dermatologists

hair

SUN PROTECTION:

Kérastase Solaire Voile Protecteur—
like a sunscreen for colored hair;
www.kerastase.com; available in
most selective hair salons

Kérastase Bain Après-Soleil Shampoo—nourishes hair after exposure to the sun, salt water, and chlorine; www.kerastase.com; available in most selective hair salons

Kérastase Solaire Waterproof Gelée—like a sunscreen for normal hair; www.kerastase.com; available in most selective hair salons

Phytotheratrie Phytoplage—"The Original" sun protection oil; www.phyto.com; 800-55PHYTO

NOURISHING HAIR PRODUCTS:

Aveda Personal Blends Shampoo—www.aveda.com; 866-823-1425; available at hair salons

Kérastase Huile Protective—www.kerastase.com; available in most selective hair salons

Kérastase Lumi-Extract—www.kerastase.com; available in most selective hair salons

Kérastase Oleo-Relax—www.kerastase.com; available in most selective hair salons

Kérastase Volumactive—www.kerastase.com; available in most selective hair salons

L'Oréal Paris ColorSpa Moisture Actif—www.lorealparisusa.com; available at drugstores

L'Oréal Paris Color VIVE and Conditioner—www.loreal parisusa.com; available at drugstores

L'Oréal Paris VIVE Fresh-Shine Shampoo and Conditioner—www.lorealparisusa.com; available at drugstores

Neutrogena Clean Color-Defending Shampoo—www.neutrogena.com; 800-582-4048; available at drugstores

Neutrogena Clean Replenishing Shampoo—www.neutrogena.com; 800-582-4048; available at drugstores

Philip B. Peppermint and Avocado Shampoo—www.philipb.com; 800-643-5556

VOLUMIZING AND HAIR THICKENING PRODUCTS:

Kérastase Volumactive Shampoo—www.kerastase.com; available in most selective hair salons

Nexxus Diametress Luscious Hair Thickening Shampoo—www.nexxus.com; 805-968-6900; available at salons

Phytocyane Thinning Hair Revitalizing Lotion—www.phyto.com; 800-55PHYTO

Privé Amplifying Shampoo—866-351-1193; available at Privé Salon

Progaine styling products—www.progaine.com; 877-PROGAINE

Rogaine for Women—www.rogaine.com/women; 800-ROGAINE

FAVORITE SALONS:

Frederic Fekkai—www.fredericfekkai.com; 15 E. 57th St., New York, NY 10022; 212-753-9500

John Frieda Salon—www.johnfrieda.com; 797 Madison Ave., New York, NY 10021; 212-879-1000

Garren New York—www.garrennewyork.com; 712 Fifth Ave., New York, NY 10019; 212-841-9400

Sally Hershberger at John Frieda—www.johnfrieda.com; 8440 Melrose Place, Los Angeles, CA 90069; 323-653-4040

Stephen Knoll—www.stephenknoll.com; 625 Madison Ave., New York, NY 10022; 212-421-0100

Louis Licari—www.louislicari.com; 693 Fifth Ave., New York, NY 10022; 212-758-2090

Pierre Michel Haute Coiffure—
www.pierremichelsalon.com;
131 E. 57th St., New York, NY
10022; 212-755-9500; visit colorist
Laura Nieu

Privé Salon—7373 Beverly Blvd.,
Los Angeles, CA 90036;
323-931-5559

HAIR TREATMENT:

The Phillip Kingsley Trichological
Centre offers cosmetic improvement
of damaged hair, thinning hair, and
hair loss, as well as treatment for
scalp problems—16 E. 53rd St.,
New York, NY 10022; 800-745-1653

principle 2:
nurture your
spirit

Michele Bernhardt, Inner World—
www.innerworldmedia.com;
212-535-4144; Michele Bernhardt is
a renowned healer and astrologer.

products:

Aura Cacia aromatherapy bath
salts—www.auracacia.co;
800-669-3275

Blue Pearl Classic Champa
incense—www.bluepearl
incense.com; 877-890-6336

Nag Champa incense—available at
yoga and spiritual bookstores

yoga resources:

Anusara Yoga, with John Friend—
www.anusara.com; 888-398-9642

Jivamukti Yoga Center—
www.jivamuktiyoga.com;
800-295-6814

Kripalu Center for Yoga and
Health—www.kripalu.org;
800-741-7353

Maha Yoga, with Steve Ross—
www.steveross.com; 310-899-0047

Om Yoga Center—
www.omyoga.com; 212-254-7884

The Omega Institute for Holistic
Studies—www.eomega.org;
800-944-1001

Piedmont Yoga Studio, with Rodney
Yee—www.piedmontyoga.com;
510-652-3336

Shambhala Parrot Cay in the
Turks and Caicos—
www.shambhalaretreat.com;
649-946-7788

Siddha Yoga Bookstore—
www.bookstore.siddhayoga.org;
888-422-3334

SYDA Foundation—
www.siddhayoga.org; 845-434-2000

Yoga Works, with Shiva Ray—
www.yogaworks.com; 310-393-5150

To find out what's going on in your
area involving yoga or yoga retreats,
pick up *Yoga Journal*. To subscribe,
visit www.yogajournal.com or call
800-600-YOGA.

books on meditation:

Autobiography of a Yogi by
Paramahansa Yogananda (Self-
Realization Fellowship, 1979).
An insider's view on the philosophy
of yoga.

The Bhaghavad Gita, translated by
Steven Mitchell (Three Rivers
Press, 2002). A literary and spiritual
masterpiece that is the core text of
the Hindu tradition, and has been
treasured by American writers from
Emerson to Thoreau.

From the Finite to the Infinite by
Swami Muktananda (SYDA
Foundation, 1994). Illuminating
questions and answers about all
phases of spiritual life.

The Heart of Meditation by Sally
Kempton/Swami Durgananda
(SYDA Foundation, 2002). A
fabulous speaker who makes
profound thought accessible, Swami
Durgananda has written a practical
guide to meditation that will
positively change the way you
meditate.

*How to Know God: The Yoga
Aphorisms of Patanjali*, translated
by Swami Prabhavananda and
Christopher Isherwood (Vedanta
Press and Bookshop, 1996). A
profound book that slowly builds on
each thought—one of my favorites.

Light on Yoga by B.K.S. Iyengar
(Schocken Books, 1995). A yoga
classic, this book is a guide to the
philosophy and practice of yoga,
including descriptions of yoga
postures and breathing exercises.

Meditate by Swami Muktananda (SYDA Foundation, 1999). A clear, step-by-step introduction to meditation by the great meditation master.

Where Are You Going? by Swami Muktananda (SYDA Foundation, 1994). An excellent introduction to spiritual life.

The Yoga of Discipline by Swami Chidvilasananda (SYDA Foundation, 1996). A guide to fully understanding and creating freedom of the five senses.

favorite meditation music:

(All available at the SYDA Yoga Bookstore—www.bookstore.siddhayoga.org)

The Bliss of Freedom—Instrumental improvisations of chants and devotional songs

The Elixir of the Saints—Indian devotional songs sung by Joyce Wells

Om Namah Shivaya (Bhupali Raga)—Chanting by Gurumayi Chidvilasananda. A classic.

Raga Taranga—Lyrical and uplifting instrumental music of Siddha Yoga

Remembrance—Piano improvisations by Kenny Warner

Samba Sadashiva—Meditative chant sung by Joyce Wells

Songs of Ecstasy—Indian devotional songs sung by Meg Christian

Tamboura—Soothing instrumental sounds that draw you inward for meditation

charities and volunteering opportunities:

You may have your own charity, but for those of you who might not know where to start, here are a few wonderful organizations I have enjoyed being involved with.

The Breast Cancer Research Foundation—www.bcrfcure.org; 866-FIND-A-CURE. Founded by Evelyn Lauder in 1993, this is the first and largest national organization dedicated solely to funding clinical and genetic research on breast cancer.

CareerPeeks Foundation—www.careerpeeks.org; 212-317-1462. This is a nonprofit educational organization primarily focused on providing insightful and interactive experiences (peeks) into a variety of career paths available to young adults between the ages of 18 and 26.

Caring for Children and Families with AIDS—call 323-931-9828 for information. Based in Los Angeles, this organization provides a home for foster children who have AIDS or are HIV-positive, counseling for families who are living with AIDS, and adoption services for children in need. My daughter, Ryan, is on its board of directors.

Civitas—www.civitas.org. Produces and distributes practical, easy-to-use tools that assist adults in making the best possible decisions on behalf of children.

Elizabeth Glaser Pediatric AIDS Foundation—www.pedaids.org; 212-448-6654. This nonprofit

organization is dedicated to identifying, funding, and conducting pediatric HIV/AIDS research—and now other serious and life-threatening diseases—affecting children.

Green Chimneys—www.greenchimneys.org; 845-279-2995. Helps children at risk by giving them the responsibility of caring for abused animals.

Look Good . . . Feel Better—www.lookgoodfeelbetter.org; 800-395-LOOK. A program that offers a makeover for the spirit, Look Good . . . Feel Better teaches cancer patients techniques to counter the appearance-related effects of cancer treatment.

The Make-A-Wish Foundation—www.wish.org; 800-722-9474. Through its wish-granting work, Make-A-Wish enriches the lives of children with life-threatening illnesses, reaching more than 97,000 children worldwide to date.

Making Waves—510-237-3434. Established in 1989, this inner-city youth education program admits children in the 5th grade and stays with them until they complete high school. A rigorous academic program, Making Waves now serves over 400 children in northern California.

MENTOR/The National Mentoring Partnership—www.mentoring.org; 703-224-2200. Connects young Americans with caring adult mentors, and provides adult volunteers with the resources to find mentoring opportunities.

The Nancy Davis Foundation for Multiple Sclerosis—www.erasems.org; 310-440-4842. Dedicated to the treatment and ultimate cure of multiple sclerosis. Their annual Race to Erase MS gala benefit has raised over $14 million to date for MS research.

The Ovarian Cancer Research Fund—www.ocrf.org; 800-873-9569. Devoted to the formulation of early diagnostic treatment programs and research toward the ultimate conquest of ovarian cancer. OCRF also supports patients and their loved ones through its various outreach programs.

Points of Light Foundation—www.pointsoflight.org; 800-VOLUNTEER. Based in Washington, D.C., Points of Light is devoted to promoting volunteerism through a network of over 500 Volunteer Centers.

The Prasad Project—www.prasad.org; 845-434-0376. Dedicated to providing services internationally for children, families, and communities in need, PRASAD has programs in the areas of medical care, dental care, nutrition, education, and community development.

Safe Horizon—www.safehorizon.org; 212-577-7700. Known for its pioneering work in domestic violence and child abuse, Safe Horizon is the nation's leading victims' assistance, advocacy, and violence protection organization.

Suited for Change—www.suitedforchange.org; 202-293-0351. Provides professional clothing and ongoing career education to low-income women in the Washington, D.C., area.

USA Weekend Magazine Make-A-Difference Day—www.usaweekend.com/diffday; 800-416-3824. This national day of helping others takes place on the fourth Saturday of October every year, and involves over 2 million volunteers helping to make a difference in their communities.

V-Day—visit www.vday.org for more information. A nonprofit corporation, founded by playwright and activist Eve Ensler, V-Day distributes funds to grassroots, national, and international organizations and programs working to stop violence against women and girls.

principle 3: honor your body

products:

Boca Foods Company—www.bocaburger.com. Boca makes a terrific line of meatless products made with organic or natural ingredients.

The Coffee Bean and Tea Leaf Vanilla Powder—www.coffeebean.com; 800-TEA-LEAF

Guayakí Yerba Maté—www.guayaki.com; 888-GUAYAKI. A powerful rejuvenating beverage grown in the rain forest.

Luna Bars—www.lunabar.com; 800-LUNABAR

SteviaPlus dietary supplement—www.steviaplus.com; 800-899-9908

markets:

True Foods Market—www.truefoodsmarket.com; 877-274-5914. An online market featuring over 1,000 of the finest natural food products, True Foods ships nationally and to over 30 countries worldwide.

Urban Organic—www.urbanorganic.com; 718-499-4321. A home-delivery organic produce service for the New York metropolitan area.

Whole Foods Markets—visit www.wholefoods.com to find a local store

exercise:

If you're having trouble finding a different way to exercise, you can try one of these:

Backroads—www.backroads.com; 800-GO-ACTIVE. "The world's #1 active travel company" offers vacations designed for active individuals who love the outdoors.

Body Trends—www.bodytrends.com; 800-549-1667. Rex Bird researches across the country for the best health and fitness products, from treadmills to workout tapes. There's a customer-support hotline that can walk you through the use of every product.

Country Walkers—www.countrywalkers.com; 800-464-9255. Offers unique walking experiences that foster an appreciation for diverse cultures and habitats around the world.

Outward Bound—www.outwardbound.com; 866-467-7651. Through its programs, including wilderness schools and expeditionary learning trips, Outward Bound helps participants develop self-reliance, responsibility, teamwork, confidence, compassion, and environmental and community stewardship.

spas:

Cal-A-Vie—www.calavie.com; 29402 Spa Havens Way, Vista, CA 92084; 866-SPAHAVENS

Canyon Ranch Health Resort—www.canyonranch.com; 800-742-9000

The Golden Door—www.goldendoor.com; P.O. Box 463077, Escondido, CA 92046; 800-424-0777

Miraval Life in Balance—www.miravalresort.com; 5000 E. Via Estancia Miraval, Catalina, AZ 85739; 800-232-3969

The Oaks at Ojai—www.oaksspa.com; 122 E. Ojai Ave., Ojai, CA 93023; 800-753-6257

Rancho la Puerta—www.rancholapuerta.com; P.O. Box 69, Tecate, CA 91980; 800-443-7565

Visit Spa Finder at www.spafinders.com or call 212-924-6800 ext. 289; a great resource for finding your ideal spa experience.

nutritionists:

Lisa Powell, M.S., R.D.—Nutrition director at Canyon Ranch Health Resort in Tucson, AZ; 520-749-9000 ext. 4284

Yvonne Nienstadt—Nutrition director for Cal-A-Vie; 760-945-2055

To find a dietitian near you, visit the American Dietetic Association website, www.eatright.org; 800-877-1600

fitness and nutrition book picks:

Ayurveda for Women: A Guide to Vitality and Health by Dr. Robert Svoboda (Inner Traditions, 2000). This guide to Ayurveda, an age-old method of healing the body, mind, and spirit, is specially geared to the unique needs of women.

The Complete Illustrated Guide to the Alexander Technique by Glynn MacDonald (Element Books, 1998). This is a step-by-step illustrated guide to this technique, which is intended to enhance posture and well-being.

Eating Well for Optimum Health by Andrew Weil, M.D. (Quill, 2001). A thorough and scientific guide to nutritious eating and a healthy lifestyle.

Fast Food Nation by Eric Schlosser (Houghton Mifflin, 2001). A fascinating exposé on the fast-food industry.

Food and Healing by Annemarie Colbin (Ballantine Books, 1996). A guide to the nutritional value of the foods we eat and how food can be used to heal.

Food and Our Bones by Annemarie Colbin (Plume, 1998). A guide to building strong bones through the foods we eat.

The Okinawa Program by Drs. Willcox, Willcox, and Suzuki (Three Rivers Press, 2002). A study of the traditional diet of Okinawa and its connection to longevity.

The Promise of Sleep by William C. Dement, M.D. (Dell, 2000). A comprehensive and interesting study of the power of sleep and the connection between sleep and longevity.

Walking Yoga by Ila Sarley and Garrett Sarley (Fireside, 2002). A wonderfully accessible program that integrates yoga principles with this most natural of exercises.

web resources:

The Alexander Technique— www.alexandertechnique.com; a comprehensive guide to Alexander Technique resources.

Mayo Clinic Health Oasis— www.mayohealth.org; provides up-to-date and useful health information, includes content for a comprehensive array of topics.

National Women's Health Information Center— www.4women.gov; a service from the federal government that provides access to a variety of women's health information resources.

Shape Up America!— www.shapeup.org; a national initiative to promote healthy weight and increased physical activity in America that provides a wealth of informative and helpful resources.

USDA guide to community-sustained agricultural programs— www.nal.usda.gov/afsic; community-sustained agricultural programs are rooted in the philosophy that communities and farmers working together can support the productivity of local farms, conserve the earth's resources, and preserve the earth's viability. These groups are successful due to their long-term commitment to local farms. Members of CSAs pay a fixed seasonal fee to share in the weekly bounty of the farmers' harvest.

USDA guide to farmers' markets—
www.ams.usda.gov/farmersmarkets;
a directory that helps you find a
farmer's market in your area.

WebMD—www.mywebmd.com; a
practical, relevant content source for
health and medicine, providing
information on a wide variety of
topics.

principle 4: discover your wisdom

lifelong learning:

92nd Street Y, New York City—
www.92ndsty.org; Lexington Ave. at
92nd St., New York, NY 10128;
212-415-5500

AARP—www.aarp.org; 601 E St.,
NW, Washington, D.C. 20049;
800-424-3410; AARP (formally
known as the American Association
of Retired Persons), is a nonprofit
membership organization dedicated
to addressing the needs and interests
of persons 50 and older.

Berlitz—www.berlitz.com;
400 Alexander Park, Princeton, NJ
08540; 609-514-9650

Fathom: The Source for Online
Learning—www.fathom.com;
330 Fifth Ave., New York, NY
10001; 877-731-6941

Institute of Culinary Education—
www.iceculinary.com; 50 W. 23rd
St., New York, NY 10010;
212-847-0770

The Learning Annex—visit
www.learningannex.com to find
a nearby program

Metropolitan Museum of Art
Travel Programs—
www.metmuseum.org/events/
ev_travel.asp; 1000 Fifth Ave., New
York, NY 10028-0198; 212-650-2110

Toastmasters International—
www.toastmasters.org; P.O. Box
9052, Mission Viejo, CA 92690;
949-858-8255

Yoga Journal Events—
www.yogajournal.com/yjevents;
2054 University Ave., Berkeley, CA
94704; 510-841-9200

good reads:

I love to recommend good books—
it's like setting up friends on a blind
date. Of course, everybody's tastes
differ, nevertheless, I still want to
share with you some of the books
I've recently read and enjoyed.
Please feel free to send me your
recommendations. I'd love to hear
from you.

A Walk with a White Bushman by
Laurens Van Der Post (William
Morrow and Co., 1987)

A Woman's Life by Guy de
Maupassant, translated by H.N.O.
Sloman (Viking Press, 1978)

The Bluest Eye by Toni Morrison
(Penguin USA, 2000)

Call It Sleep by Henry Roth
(Noonday Press, 1992)

Girl With a Pearl Earring by Tracy
Chevalier (E. P. Dutton, 1999)

*It's Only Too Late If You Don't Start
Now: How to Create Your Second
Life at Any Stage* by Barbara Sher
(Delacorte Press, 1999)

Life Makeovers by Cheryl
Richardson (Broadway Books, 2000)

Monkeys by Susan Minot (Vintage
Books, 2000)

Nana by Emile Zola, translated by
George Holden (Viking Press, 1972)

*Nonzero: The Logic of Human
Destiny* by Robert Wright
(Pantheon Books, 1999)

The Piano Tuner by Daniel Mason
(Knopf, 2002)

The Pilot's Wife by Anita Shreve
(Back Bay Books, 1999)

Promiscuities by Naomi Wolf
(Fawcett Books, 1998)

The Red and the Black by Stendhal,
translated by Roger Gard (Penguin,
2002)

A Return to Love by Marianne
Williamson, (HarperCollins, 1996)

She by Robert A. Johnson
(HarperCollins, 1989)

A Short Guide to a Happy Life by
Anna Quindlen (Random House,
2000)

The Spiritual Heritage of India by
Swami Prabhavananda (Vedanta
Press and Bookshop, 1979)

Stand Up for Your Life: Develop the Courage, Confidence, and Character to Fulfill Your Greatest Potential by Cheryl Richardson (Free Press, 2002)

Suze Orman's Financial Guidebook by Suze Orman (Three Rivers Press, 2002)

The Wisdom of Menopause by Christiane Northrup, M.D. (Bantam Doubleday, 2003)

The Wonder of Girls by Michael Gurian (Pocket Star, 2002)

principle 5: stay connected

Lynda P. Haddon— www.multiplebirthsfamilies.com; Lynda's site contains a wealth of information for families expecting twins, triplets, and more. In addition, it provides bereavement support for families who have lost multiple-birth babies.

favorite restaurants:

The Garden Market—3811 Santa Claus La., Carpenteria, CA 93013; 805-745-5505

Il Gattopardo—33 W. 54th St., New York, NY 10019; 212-246-0412

Il Ristorante di Giorgio Baldi— 114 W. Channel Rd., Santa Monica Canyon, CA 90402; 310-573-1660

Milos—125 W. 55th St., New York, NY 10019; 212-245-7400

Osteria del Circo—120 W. 55th St., New York, NY 10019; 212-265-3636

Pane e Vino—1482 E. Valley Rd., Montecito, CA 93108; 805-969-9274

Trattoria Mollie—1250 Coast Village Rd., Montecito, CA 93108; 805-565-9381

Via Quadronno—25 E. 73rd St., New York, NY 10021; 212-650-9880

Resource Guide

Index

AARP, 246

AARP: The Magazine, 246

acne, 52, 53, 55, 56

adventure (the), 1–17
   pursuing, 305–09

age, xviii, 20–21, 36
   appreciating, 209–10
   grace and strength of, 306
   lying about, 313

Age Quake, The, 4–9

Ageless Living, xvii, 19, 20, 21

ageless living dialogue, 311–18

Ageless Living Principles, xx,
   19–23, 210, 258, 306,
   308, 309

aging, graceful, 307–08

aging process, 19, 21, 163,
   208–09
   breathing and, 49
   changing concept of, 5
   new definition of, 212
   pull of, 38
   and skin, 46–47, 65

alcohol, 48–49, 54

Alexander Technique, 38–39

aloe vera, 71

alpha-hydroxy acids (AHA),
   64–65

American Academy of
   Dermatology, 56

Angelo, Fra, 127

Annunciation (artwork), 127

antioxidants, 149, 163, 173

appearance, 36, 37, 145
   taking care of, 258

apricots, dried, 149

Archive of Internal Medicine,
   The, 269

art, spirit of, 126–28

asparagus, 148

Ativan, 195

attitude, 87, 213, 317
   affects experience, 134
   and exercise, 193–94

Aura Cacia Tranquility (bath
   salts), 131

awareness, 102, 215, 216, 217,
   218
   acting with, 258
   of what you are eating, 176,
   177

baby-boomer women, 5, 6

Baptiste, Baron, 295

bath rituals, 131–32

beans, 148

beauty, 128, 312
   healthy, 184
   radiates from us, 35–36
   true, 7, 26

beauty and fashion industry,
   5–6, 7–9, 314

beauty bottle basics, 57–60t

beauty products, 37, 87–88

beauty rituals, 32

bedtime rituals, 198–99

beta-carotene, 148, 149, 150,
   151

bike riding, 125–26

birthdays, 297–99

blackstrap molasses, 148

Boca Foods, 164

body, 42, 145, 146
   balance and alignment of,
   39
   care of, 141–42

changing, 41
   healthy, well-cared-for, 27,
   200
   honoring, 139–201
   needs for health, 147–96
   wisdom of, 228–34

body types, 184

bonds, blessed, 274–77

bone mass/density, 191, 195,
   202

bones, 155–56, 194–96

book groups, 247–48

breasts, heavy, and posture, 41

breathing, 133–35

brewer's yeast, 148

broccoli, 149

brown rice, 148

butterfly effect, 268–74

caffeine, 49, 172–73

calcium, 41, 149, 151, 155–57,
   195–96
   sources of, 150, 157

cancer, 201

cantaloupe, 149

carbohydrates, 152

carrots, 149

celebrations, 286–88

Centers for Disease Control
   and Prevention (CDC),
   184

challenges, xvii, xviii, xix,
   15–16, 31–32
   as gifts, 16, 215
   meeting, xx

change, xvii, 1
   at midlife, 10

Chaos Theory, 268

Chidvilasananda, Swami, 119, 180
choices, 3, 9, 21–22
  for body, 144–45
  in food, 169–70
  in midlife, 229
  in nurturing spirit, 94
cholesterol, 160, 164
chromium, 148, 150
Clé de Peau Beauté Masque Transparence, 71
cleansing (skin), 60–66
  basics, 60–62
  supplemental, 63–64
closure, 220
CNN, 8
coffee, 172–73
Coliseum, 127
collagen, 50, 53, 71
coloring hair, 78, 81–85
  tips for, 84–85
coming together, 288–90
community
  connecting to, 231
  importance of, 264
  links to, 258–59
  reaching out to, 257–304
  resources in, 295
  sense of, 266, 268
  sense of, and health, 259–61
  volunteering in, 293–94
complex carbohydrates, 157–58
  sources of, 158
conditioners, 78–79
connection, loss of, 259
connection to nature, 96
connection to others 100–01, 241, 257–304
  book groups, 247–48
  circle of, 258–64
connection with living things, 93, 94–95, 96, 98–99
conscious breathing, 133–35

conscious eating, 176–78
conscious living, 214–15, 306
contemplation, 111, 112, 113, 121
  great art, 126
  through journaling, 223–24, 226
copper, 150
copper peptides, 71
cortisol, 51, 52
cosmetic surgery, 317–18
cosmetics, 36, 57–60
  see also beauty products
courage, 14, 32, 237
Crème de la Mer, 66, 74
Culinary Institute (New York), 169, 298–99

dance, 192
David (artwork), 126–27
deep breathing, 44–45
  and skin, 49
dehydration, 49, 166
  skin, 52–53
depression, 28, 260–61
dermatologist, 54–57, 74, 86
diabetes, 201
diet, 41
  balanced, 88
  healthful, 145
diets, 157, 184
digestion, 160, 177
Discover Your Wisdom (principle), 23, 205–55, 258, 306
  resource guide, 336–37
doing for others, 290–91
dry skin, 54

e-mail, 278, 279, 284, 285
Early Show, The, 9
eating
  consciously, 176–78
  replacing bad habits with good, 172–75

eating well, 144, 146–83
education, continuing, 241–43, 245–46
effect we have on others, 268–74
effort, 255
  value of, 237–39
elastin, 50, 53
Elgin Marbles, 127
endorphins, 189
energy, 2, 13, 133, 163
  creating, 139–201
environment
  and skin, 46, 50, 54
Estée Lauder, 8
  Advanced Night Repair, 66
estrogen, 53, 163
Evans, Lydia, 56–57
events, 295–96
evolution, 21, 23, 209, 210
  challenges gift for, 215
exercise, 41–42, 88, 142, 145, 183–96
  adventure of, 187–90
  outdoors, 124, 126
  and posture, 40
  sneaking into busy day, 190–91
  types of, 191–94
exfoliants, 63–64, 87
  how to pick, 64–65
experience(s), 2, 207
  accumulated, 206, 228, 229
  drawing on, 205–55
  new, 239
  tuning in to lessons of, 258
  value in, 317
extended families, role in, 10

fad diets, 157
family, 231
  links to, 258–59
  reaching out to, 257–304
family outings, 302
farmers' markets, 168

Index

Fathom, 245
fats, 152
   healthy/unhealthy, 158–59
   sources of, 159*t*
fear of unknown, 209
fiber, 148, 149, 150, 157
   sources of, 160
Fields, Kathy, 55–56
flavonoids, 161–62
flaxseed, 149
folic acid, 148, 151
   sources of, 160
food(s), 145, 146–47
   and exercise, 42
   joy and celebration of,
      178–83
   seasonal, fresh, organic,
      166–69
   and skin, 50
   variety in, 169–70
Forever Angels (newsletter),
   276
forgiveness, 220
Fossey, Dian, 211
fractures, osteoporosis-related,
   195–96
free radicals, 47, 51
French Deluxe Vanilla
   Powder, 173
Frick Museum, 122–23
friends, 231
   bonds with, 276–77
   links to, 258–59
   reaching out to, 257–304
   reconnecting with, 300–01
future
   connection to, 264–66
   journaling and, 227

gardening, 119–21
Garren (hairstylist), 83
generations, connecting across,
   265, 266
giving, 102
   acts of, 303–04

finding spirit through,
   113–15
God, 127
   connection with, 93, 95
   partnership with, 239
Gogh, Vincent van, 127
golfing, 125
Good Housekeeping, 295
Goodall, Jane, 211
grace, 238–39
gratitude, 135–37, 214, 239,
   316–17
gravity, 19, 38, 39
   effect on skin, 46
green tea, 173
greens, 150
growing up, 207–08
Guayakí Yerba Maté, 173

habits
   skin care, 47–53
habits (eating)
   replacing bad with good,
      172–75
hair, 77–89
   changing style, 80
   trimming, 79–80
hair appointment, 44
hair loss, 85–86
hair thickening products,
   86
Hamilton, Carol, 80, 283
happiness, xviii, xix, 235
Harvard Nurses' Health Study,
   196
healing, 220, 221, 275–76
health, 2, 139–201
Health (magazine), 295
healthy body, needs for,
   147–66
healthy eating, seven steps to,
   147–83
heart disease, 184, 201
helping others, 274–76
hiking, 192, 301–02

holding patterns, 214–21,
   223–26
Honor Your Body (principle),
   23, 139–201, 258, 306
   resource guide, 332–36
How to Know God (Patanjali),
   129
humidifier, 72
hyaluronic acids, 71
hydration, 66, 88

Il Gattopardo (restaurant),
   266–68, 298
incense, 107, 129
inner life, 27
   developing, 91–137
insight(s), 216, 221, 238
interests, sharing, 294–97
intimacy, 229, 233
irritant acne, 50
isoflavones, 195
isolation, 259
isopropyl alcohol, 63

Jordan, Barbara, 211
journaling, 121, 221–28, 316
Just Ask a Woman (co.), 11

Kail, Donna, 283
Kérastase Bain Après-Soleil
   Shampoo, 85
Kérastase Huile Protective, 85
Kérastase Lumi-Extract, 79
Kérastase Oleo-Relax, 79
Kérastase products, 79
Kérastase Solaire Voile
   Protecteur, 85
Kérastase Volumactive, 86
kindness, random acts of,
   302–04

La Roche-Posay Active C, 71
La Roche-Posay Anthélios, 74
Lancôme Hydra-Intense
   Masque, 71

Lancôme Primordial Intense, 66
Lancôme Vitabolic, 71
language(s), learning new, 248–49
Lauder, Leonard, 283
learning, 240–41, 243
Learning Annex, 245
Lelouch, Claude, 125–26, 265–66
Licari, Louis, 81, 83
life
    is arc, 204, 311
    changing, 1, 3
    claiming, 9–13
    good, happy, xix
    is miracle, 93–94
    take control of, 235
life force (Shakti), 94, 179
lifestyle, healthy, 48
lignans, 149
live large and true, 98–101
live true, 2–4, 19, 207
    see also true life
longevity, connection and, 259–60
Look Your Best (principle), 23, 25–89, 258, 306, 312–13
    cosmetic surgery in, 317–18
    exercise in, 41–42
    resource guide, 321–27
look-your-best checklist, 87–89
L'Oréal Paris, 8–9, 283
L'Oréal Paris Age Perfect Day Cream, 66
L'Oréal Paris Age Perfect Night Cream, 66
L'Oréal Paris ColorSpa Moisture Actif, 83
L'Oréal Paris FUTUR.e Moisturizer Normal to Oily, 66
L'Oréal Paris Color VIVE , 78
L'Oréal Paris VIVE Fresh-Shine, 78

losses, 19, 209
love, 99, 258
love the one you're with, 34–37
low point(s), 272–73
Lufkin, Dan, 283

magazines, 295–96
magnesium, 148, 151
Make-A-Wish, 293
Making Waves, 293
manicure, 43
massage, 44
meals, 178, 182–83
    regular, 171
    see also food(s)
media, 213, 314, 315
    celebrate youth, 208
medical checkups, 200, 203t
meditation, 44, 104, 106–13, 121, 316
    breathing in, 133–34
memories, creating, 285
menopause, 53, 80, 213
metabolism, 41
Metropolitan Museum of Art, 251
Michelangelo, 126–27
midlife, xx, 1–2, 3–4, 7, 8, 14, 87, 309
    accumulated experiences in, 206
    beauty at, 26–27, 36
    body at, 140–41, 142–43
    change in, xvii, 10, 317
    continuing education in, 241–42
    exercise in, 184–87
    fulfilling our dreams at, 255
    gateway to second half of life, 314
    gifts of, 134
    giving at, 113
    and gratitude, 136
    and habits, 172

hair care in, 80
letting go of patterns, 216, 220
love of body in, 187
meaning in life, 99–100
myths and maxims, 319t
new responsibilities in, 316
nutritional needs at, 178
opportunities in, 112–13
outlook in, 111–12
owning our desires in, 232
picking up threads in life, 235
posture at, 38
questions at, 9–10
relationship problems in, 278
rituals at, 130
search for meaning, 315
sex at, 229–30
skin at, 48
and sleep, 197
spirituality at, 92–93, 106
transitions in, 21–22
wisdom at, 112
wisdom for wisdom's sake, 245
women as pioneers, 212–14
women at, 307, 309
midlife maintenance, 200–03
minerals, 150, 152, 169
mistakes, admitting, 219–20
misunderstandings, 279–80
moisturizers, daytime/nighttime, 66
moisturizing
    basic, 65–66
Monet, Claude, 127
More Magazine, 295–96
movement
    sneaking into busy day, 190–91
    and spirit, 123–26
moving forward, 220
Multiple Births Canada, 276

music, 117–19, 121–22
Mustela sunsticks, 74

Natura Bissé, 74
nature, 145
    communing with, 124–25,
      126
    is nurture, 95–98
    oneness with, 120–21
    sounds in, 119
    spending time in, 104
    walking in, 124–25
needs, giving voice to, 233–34
neighborhood restaurant,
    266–68
Neutrogena
    SPF 45 sunblock, 74
Neutrogena Clean Color-
    Defending shampoo, 78
Neutrogena Clean
    Replenishing, 78
New York City, 261–63
Nexxus, 86
92nd Street Y (NYC), 295
nourishing basics (skin), 67–70t
nourishing skin, 60, 65–66,
    67–70t
    supplemental, 71–72
nurture, nature is, 95–98
Nurture Your Spirit
    (principle), 23, 91–137,
    258, 306
    resource guide, 327–32
nutrition
    what we need every day,
      152, 153–55t
nuts, 150

O: The Oprah Magazine, 223,
    295
oats, 150
oily skin, 54
Okinawa, Japan, 259–60, 292
omega-3 fatty acids, 149, 151,
    158, 159

sources of, 161
omega-6 fats, 159
One-to-One, 293
oneness, 99, 119
opening yourself to
    possibility(ies), 35, 230
opportunities, 213–14
    for connection, 296, 297
    expand with age, 214
    for kindness, 302
    in midlife, 112–13
osteoporosis, 156–57, 194–95,
    202
    risk for, 152
overwashing (skin), 50–51

pampering ourselves, 43–44
papaya, 150
parents, responsibility as, 10
Parthenon, 127
passion(s)
    adventures supporting, 305
    in connection, 291
    following, 239–40, 241
    power of, 234–37
passport(s), 249–51
past (the), connection to,
    264–66
Patanjali (sage), 102, 129–30
patterns, 214–21, 223–26, 237
    recognizing, 217–18
pedicure, 43
Philip B. Peppermint and
    Avocado shampoo, 78
phone call(s), 284
physical transitions
    at midlife, 142–43
phytochemicals, 161–62
    sources of, 162t
Phytocyane, 86
phytoestrogens, 163
Phytoplage, 85
Pierce, Rusty, 283
Pietà (artwork), 127
pilates, 40, 193

Points of Light, 293
position yourself, 37–41
posture, 37–41
    while walking, 42
potassium, 148, 149, 150, 151
potential
    power of, 13–16
    realizing, 19
prana (energy)
    see energy
pranayama breathing, 44, 135
premature aging, 51, 73
prescription drugs
    and loss of bone density,
      195
Prisoners, The (artwork), 127
Privé Amplifying Shampoo, 86
Proactiv Solution, 55–56
problem solving, 92–93, 101,
    104, 312
processed foods, 147–48
Progaine, 86
protection (skin), 60, 72–77
protein, 150, 152, 163–64
prunes, 150
Psychology and Aging, 261
pursuits, 294–97

quiet place, 107–08
Quinlan, Mary Lou, 10–12

Ray, Shiva, 295
reach out and touch, 283–86
reading, 246–48
red pepper, 151
Redbook, 295
redwoods, 97–98
relationships, 100, 145, 228,
    259
    changing, 21
    difficulties in, 277–82
    passion in, 235
    reaching out in, 284–85
resignation, 4, 13
resistance exercises, 191

resource guide, 321–38
respect yourself, 27–30, 38
responsibilities, new, 316
rest, 144, 196–99
retinoids, 64–65
reunions, 299–301
Richardson, Cheryl, xiii–xv,
    227–28
ricotta cheese, 151
Rit Sun Guard Laundry
    Treatment, 77
rituals, 121, 128–30
    bath, 131–32
    bedtime, 198–99
Rodan, Katie, 55–56
Rogaine, 86
role models, 212, 308
romantic relationships, 231–34
Roosevelt, Eleanor, 211
rosacea, 48, 50, 52, 55
Royal Edinburgh Hospital, 41
Rudolph, Wilma, 211
rule of three, 59–77

sacred spaces, 121–23
sadhana, 128
salmon, 151
Sarley, Garrett, 124, 295
Sarley, Ila, 124, 295
scents, 107, 108
scrubs and grains, 65
Sea & Ski, 74
self, gift of, 115
    see also true self
self-confidence, 32
sense of self, 32
September 11 terrorist attack,
    261–63
service, xviii
    living life as, 276
sex, 41, 228–30, 233
shampoo, 78, 85
    dandruff, 86
Shaw, George Bernard, 265
Shiseido, 74

Shriver, Deb, 283
simple carbs, 157
Sistine Chapel, 127
sitting
    posture, 40
skin, 41, 42, 45–77, 87
    color change, 82
skin cancer, 73
skin-care routine, three-step,
    59–77
skin type, 53–57
    nourishing basics, 67–70t
sleep, 88, 196–99
    and skin, 51
smoking, and skin, 51
soap, 61
soy, 151, 163, 195
spider veins, 48
spirit, 145
    in art, 126–28
    finding through giving,
        113–15
    and movement, 123–26
    nurturing, 91–137
spirit of place, 266–68
spirituality, 92–95, 106,
    129–30
    beauty and, 26–27
    neglecting, 105
Starry Night (artwork), 127
Stay Connected (principle), 23,
    257–304
    how to, 282–304
    past/present/future,
        264–66
    resource guide, 338
Steinem, Gloria, 211
SteviaTabs Stevia Extract, 173
strength, creating, 139–201
stress, 43–45, 49, 103, 104
    and breathing, 134
    causing insomnia, 198
    and posture, 40
    and skin, 52
Stryker, Rod, 295

Suited for Change, 223
sun
    skin damage, 51, 52
sun protection (skin), 72–77
    basic, 72–74
    SPF, 72, 73, 74, 76
    supplemental, 77
sun protection basics, 75
sunblock, 72–74, 75t, 76
    hair, 85
Super Foods, 148–52
sweet potatoes/yams, 151
swimming, 192

tai chi, 113–17, 192
taking care of ourself, 28, 34,
    315, 316
taking responsibility, 220, 232
talents, hidden, 246
    discovering, 252–55
telephone, 285
thanks, giving, 135–37
thinking, 19, 107
thinning hair, 85–86
thyroid, 52
time, 208
    lack of, 102–03, 105
    with loved ones, 285–86
    for self-care, 315–16
    for yourself, 91–137, 312
Toastmasters, 245
toning (skin), 60–66
    basic, 62–63
traditions, birthday, 297
trampolines, 191
transitions, 307
    midlife, 21–22
travel, 249–51
true life, xviii, 3, 13, 14, 22, 26,
    232, 237, 306
    journey toward, 309
    nurturing from living, 93
    patterns and, 217
    sex in, 229
true self, 14, 216

presenting, 25–89
trying new things, 238–55
tuning in, 101–05
turning inward, 104–05, 106

unconscious behavior, 218, 237
Upanishad, 180
UpStage, 62
UVA/UVB protection, 52, 76, 77, 87

Valium, 195
vegetarians, 163–64
Vinci, Leonardo da, 127
vitamin B, 151
vitamin B$_6$, 148
vitamin C, 50, 71, 148, 149, 150, 151
vitamin D, 195
vitamin E, 50, 152
vitamins, 152, 169
volumizing products, 86
Volunteer Center(s), 293

volunteering, 291–93
    in community, 293–94

walking, 41, 42, 43, 88
    in nature, 96–97, 124–25
    and posture, 40
Walking Yoga (Sarley and Sarley), 124
water, 165, 166
    and skin, 52–53
Water Lilies (artwork), 127
way in, the, 106–37
weight-bearing exercises, 191
weight loss, 171
wheat bran, 151
wheat germ, 152
whole foods, 147–48, 152
Whole Foods Market, 167
willpower, 188–89
Wing Chun, 186–87
wisdom, 1, 2, 3, 16, 145, 313
    of body, 228–34
    developing, 239

discovering, 205–55, 258, 306
getting in touch with, 221, 222
in midlife, 112, 245
uncovering, 210–11
yoga and, 132
witch hazel, 63
women
    pioneers, 211–14
    power of, 314–15
women over forty, 5, 6–7, 8, 311

Yee, Rodney, 295
yoga, 104, 121, 132–35, 295
    and posture, 40
Yoga Journal, 251, 295
Yoga of Discipline, The (Chidvilasananda), 180
yogurt, fat-free, 149
your best you, 30–34
Yuimaru, 260, 292

Thank you for giving me the opportunity to share this book with you. I hope it is uplifting and helpful to you in your life. Please keep in touch. You can reach me at dayle@dayle.com or visit me at www.dayle.com.